271

Current Topics in Microbiology and Immunology

Springer
Berlin
Heidelberg
New York
Barcelona
Hong Kong
London
Milan
Paris
Tokyo

T. M. KOEHLER (Ed.)

Anthrax

With 14 Figures

Springer

THERESA M. KOEHLER, Ph.D.

Department of Microbiology and Molecular Genetics,
University of Texas – Houston Medical School,
6431 Fannin Street, JFB 1.765, Houston, TX 77030, USA
e-mail: Theresa.M.Koehler@uth.tmc.edu

Cover Illustration:
Crystallographic structure of a SDS-resistant PA_{63} heptamer that may represent a prepore conformation of the protective antigen component of anthrax toxin (R. J. Collier, Harvard Medical School, Boston, MA). A phase micrograph of Bacillus anthracis cells and spores is shown in the background (E. Saile, University of Texas – Houston Medical School, Houston, TX).

ISSN 0070-217X
ISBN 3-540-43497-6
Springer-Verlag Berlin Heidelberg New York

Library of Congress Catalog Card Number 72-152360

Springer-Verlag Berlin Heidelberg New York
a member of BertelsmannSpringer Science+Business Media GmbH

http://www.springer.de

Typesetting: Fotosatz-Service Köhler GmbH, Würzburg
Cover Design: Design & Production GmbH, Heidelberg
Printed on acid-free paper SPIN: 10718427 27/3020 5 4 3 2 1 0

Preface

Bacillus anthracis is at once a microorganism of intriguing biology and historical significance. Since the pioneering work of Robert Koch and Louis Pasteur, strides in *B. anthracis* research have been matched with historical and political events. Devastating natural outbreaks of anthrax in domestic animals in Europe in the late 1800's instigated the groundbreaking investigations of early microbiologists. A surge in anthrax research during World War II resulted from the perception that *B. anthracis* could be used as an effective bioweapon. Following the Biological Weapons Convention of 1972, active research waned until the accidental release of virulent *B. anthracis* spores from a Soviet military research facility in 1979. The current human cases of inhalation and cutaneous anthrax in the United States associated with intentional release of spores are likely to lead to another wave of intense study.

Although such events have clearly provided impetus for studies of *B. anthracis*, the unique biology of this microorganism is enough to stimulate investigation. *B. anthracis* is closely-related to common soil bacteria, some disease-causing and some nonpathogenic, yet it is uniquely adapted for survival and multiplication in mammalian hosts. Typically, the infectious form of *B. anthracis* is the dormant spore. Once inside the host, this developmental bacterium germinates, becoming a vegetative organism that replicates freely in the bloodstream and other body tissues, synthesizing the anthrax toxin proteins and an antiphagocytic capsule.

From the survival of spores inside phagocytic cells during the early stages of infection, to the specific effects of the toxin proteins on eukaryotic cells and the cellular response, the relationships between *B. anthracis* and the host provide an exciting system for study of host-pathogen interactions. The presence of a secreted toxin in the serum of infected guinea pigs was first reported by Smith and Stanley in the 1950's. In recent years there has been a virtual explosion in knowledge of the biochemistry of the unique anthrax toxin proteins. The role of protective antigen, both as the facilitator for anthrax toxin entry into eukaryotic cells and as an immunogen in the human anthrax vaccine is a particularly active area of investigation. Less well-studied, but just as interesting, is the biosynthesis of the poly-D-glutamic acid capsule, again unique among capsulated bacteria. Recently, the genetic basis for the unique biology of the bacterium has received much attention. The major genetic distinction between *B. anthracis* and other closely-related *Bacillus* species is the presence of two large plasmids that carry the toxin and capsule genes. However, physiological differences between *B. anthracis* and these species cannot be fully explained by plasmid content.

This volume aims to serve as a broad survey of the biology of the *Bacillus anthracis* and the pathogenesis of anthrax disease. Early chapters provide an overview of the history of the disease, anthrax ecology and epidemiology, and the implications for evolution of the organism. Subsequent chapters include information regarding existing vaccines and those in development, synthesis and function of the anthrax toxin proteins, novel surface structures of the bacterium, macrophage interactions, and finally, genetics and virulence gene regulation. It is my hope that the volume will not only serve as a valuable reference for microbiologists with an interest in anthrax, but will motivate new investigators to join in the pursuit of answers to the many open questions regarding the biology of this fascinating microbe.

T. M. Koehler

List of Contents

List of Contributors

CHAPTER 1

Introduction: Anthrax History, Disease and Ecology

P. C. B. TURNBULL

Abstract. The familiarity with the ancient disease anthrax from the second millennium B.C. through the second millennium A.D. is reviewed, providing the backdrop to the modern understanding of this disease as covered in the remainder of the volume. By means of an overview of the aetiology, ecology, epidemiology, clinical manifestations, pathology and bacteriology of the naturally acquired disease, this opening chapter also lays down the groundwork for the subsequent state-of-the-art chapters.

1 The Disease and Its History

Anthrax is a peracute, acute or subacute disease primarily affecting herbivores but also encountered in other mammals, including humans, and occasionally birds. The word 'anthrax' is derived from the Greek *anthrakos*, meaning coal, referring to the characteristic eschar in the

P. C. B. TURNBULL
Arjemptur Technology Ltd., c/o 86 St Mark's Avenue, Salisbury SP1 3DW, UK,
Email: peterturnbull@tesco.net.

human cutaneous form of the disease. The familiar name 'black bane' and the French and Italian names for the disease, *charbon* and *carbonchio*, similarly reflect this manifestation. Names in other languages and older English names refer to other of its significant manifestations or to its sources of infection, viz *Milzbrand* (German) and *miltvuur* (Dutch), meaning 'spleen fire', *pustula maligna* (Spanish), Bradford disease, woolsorter's disease, ragpicker's disease and so on. Its numerous synonyms in many national languages and local dialects reflect the historical familiarity with the different syndromes before it was realised that they were manifestations of one etiological agent, *Bacillus anthracis* (so named by Cohn in 1875).

The antiquity of the disease has frequently caught the imagination of authors with a historical bent and its history has been extensively reviewed (Hutyra and Marek 1922; Wilson and Miles 1946; Klemm and Klemm 1959; Choquette and Broughton 1981; Dirckx 1981; Hambleton et al. 1984; Christie 1987; Turnbull 1998) Usually mentioned is that the fifth or the fifth and sixth plagues of Egypt in the time of Moses (ca. 1250 B.C.) are thought by some to have represented the earliest historical reports of the anthrax, due respectively to systemic and cutaneous forms of the disease. Anthrax appears to have featured in Asia Minor at the time of the Siege of Troy (ca. 1200 B.C.) and descriptions of the typical symptoms in the writings of Homer (ca. 1000 B.C.), Hippocrates (ca. 400 B.C.), Varro (116–27 B.C.), Virgil (70–19 B.C.) and Galen (ca. 200 A.D.) indicate that the Greeks and Romans were well acquainted with it. The disease also featured in very early Hindu literature of around 500 B.C. Records in post-Roman Europe begin with references to what is likely to have been anthrax in the 'Hippiatrika', a tenth century collection of veterinary writings, and the eleventh century 'The Medicine of Quadrupeds'. Major episodes were also recorded in 996 and 1090 in France, in 1552, 1898 and 1613–17 in Italy, in 1709–1714 in England, Germany, Hungary and Poland, in 1745–1747 in England and Holland, in the early 1800s in Russia, Holland and England, and in again in Russia the mid-1800s (Cole 1847; Salmon 1896; Wilson and Miles 1946; Klemm and Klemm 1959). In America anthrax was first reported in animals in the early 1700s (Brachman 1991) and by 1847, the description of 'bloody murrain' (Cole 1847) suggests that anthrax was well recognised under that name, and this record even includes allegedly successful vaccination of cows with 'the *vaccine virus* (pus)'.

Scientific, as opposed to historical, reports began with the descriptions of malignant pustule by Maret in 1752, Dym in 1769 and Fournier in 1769 and the description of the disease in animals by Chabert in 1780 (Wilson and Miles 1946). As summarised by Turnbull (1998), the nineteenth century saw anthrax as the first disease of man and animals shown to be caused by a microorganism and as the disease on which much of the original work on bacteria and vaccines was done. It was from studies on anthrax that many of the well-known principles of pathogenic microbiology were derived. Particularly notable milestones were: (a) the demonstration of the infectiousness of the disease by Berthelemy in 1823, Eilert in 1836 and others in the 1850s; (b) the demonstration by Davaine in 1863–64 of its transmissibility and the demonstration by Tiegel and Klebs in 1864 that the infectivity of infectious material was lost on filtration through clay filters; (c) the first observation of the bacillus by Delafond in 1838; (d) the recognition between 1860 and 1880 that the single agent could produce different manifestations ranging from malignant pustule to woolsorter's disease; (e) the formulation by Robert Koch of his famous postulates in 1877 in proving that *Bacillus anthracis* was the cause of anthrax; and (f) Pasteur's well-known pioneering work on vaccines in 1881 (Wilson and Miles 1946; Klemm and Klemm 1959; Choquette and Broughton 1981; Parvizpour 1978).

De Vos (de Vos and Turnbull 2000) has researched fascinating literature and anecdotes on anthrax among the records of early historians, explorers and travellers in nineteenth century southern Africa. Alexander in 1838 described a blood sickness in the Orange River region, Cape Province. 'Sheep occasionally get this, which is a corrupted state of the blood; the natives then kill them, and strange to say, eat them. The disease is very often communicated to those partaking of the impure flesh; and it appears in angry sores on the arms and on other parts of the body. It is very difficult to cure'. Missionary Robert Moffat in 1842 appears to be the first to chronicle the disease in a human of European descent in southern Africa, describing the disease as particularly prevalent in humans and livestock of the indigenous tribes in the north-eastern Cape Province: *'a disease which appears to be endemial, which assumes the form of a carbuncle, and carries off many cattle, and as the natives will on no account abstain from eating the dead meat, they are often attacked by it. If it happens to be near a vital part it is very frequently fatal; if internal and not suppurating outwardly it is always so. The meat of the goat which has died of this disease is particularly noxious, and I have known persons after having eaten it, cut off in five days. It is always accompanied by considerable swelling attended with great stupor, though with comparatively little pain.'* Dr. Andrew Smith, Director of an 'Expedition for Exploring Central Africa', which took place in 1834–1836, described the clinical form of anthrax in humans and domestic animals naming the disease 'bloodzichte' or 'quatsie'. In 1857 the famous explorer David Livingstone reported a very virulent disease which he called 'horse-sickness'; this from his descriptions, was undoubtedly anthrax. Probably the first to describe it in wild animals, he states that *'great numbers also of zebras are found dead with masses of foam at the nostrils, exactly as occurs in the common horse-sickness. The production of the malignant carbuncle ... by the flesh when eaten, is another proof of the disease of the tame and wild being identical'.*

These early observations on anthrax in southern Africa indicate that the disease occurred in a region that now incorporates the north-eastern part of the Cape Province and the adjoining parts of western Transvaal, Botswana and Lesotho. They also indicate a high degree of familiarity on the part of the indigenous people with the disease, suggesting its existence before the arrival of the first Europeans. This is, perhaps, in line with the description of this region of the globe as the cradle of anthrax (Smith et al. 1999). In fact anthrax was regarded as relatively insignificant in South Africa in the first decade of the twentieth century, but by 1923–1924 the disease had become markedly more prevalent, with an estimated 30,000 to 60,000 animals dying of it in 1923 (Sterne 1967). This led to the signal development in South Africa by Sterne of his successful live spore vaccine (Sterne 1937), which went on to render anthrax a controllable disease worldwide. This and analogous counterparts in China and the former USSR remain the livestock vaccines in use throughout the world today (Turnbull et al. 1998).

Programs today aimed at improved therapy and prophylaxis for anthrax still fall back on invaluable information on mortality rates of cutaneous and inhalation anthrax to be found in well-kept records in at-risk industrial processes in the early part of the twentieth century, well before treatment and vaccination were available. For example, the records of the woollen industry in the United Kingdom (Anon 1918) show that from 1896 through 1917 there were 537 external cases reported with 58 deaths (10.4%) and 56 internal cases with 55 deaths (98.2%). 'External' anthrax would undoubtedly have been what is now termed 'cutaneous' anthrax, and, being records of the woollen industry, it is almost certainly legitimate to equate 'internal' with 'inhalational'.

Although the natural disease in animals and humans declined from around 1940 through the combined application of livestock vaccines and improved veterinary and public health, the focus on anthrax took a new and somewhat sinister direction, with the next significant milestone in the history of anthrax being the upsurge in interest in it as a potential agent for biological aggression. Its earliest planned use in this context appears to have been during World War I (WHEELIS 1999) A particular incident, 'a piece of sugar containing anthrax bacilli, found in the luggage of Baron Otto Karl von Rosen, when he was apprehended in Karasjok in January 1917, suspected of espionage and sabotage' has been recalled recently (REDMOND et al. 1998). This chapter in the organism's history really began in earnest, however, with intelligence reports in World War II that Germany was developing a biological weapons capability, which, in fact, appears not to have been the case (GEISSLER 1999). However, it led directly to the notorious anthrax trials by the British in 1942–43 on Gruinard Island, off the northwest coast of Scotland, which were carried out in response to the perceived need for a practical assessment of the feasibility and hazards of biological warfare (CARTER and PEARSON 1999). Feasibility research continued in Porton Down in the United Kingdom and Fort Detrick in the United States after the war, becoming wholly defensive at the end of the 1950s in Britain (CARTER, 1992) and at the end of the 1960s in the United States when then-President Nixon renounced all biological weapons capability (CARTER and BALMER, 1999). The emphasis as far as anthrax was concerned then switched almost entirely to the pathogenesis of the disease, with the development of effective prophylaxis being the declared aim.

Although the search for a toxin on which to target vaccine-induced protection against anthrax began as early as 1889, it was military interest that brought about the veritable explosion of research which took place from the end of World War II until about 1967 and resulted not only in elucidation of the three-component nature of the anthrax toxin but also in the design and production of both the US and UK human anthrax vaccines. The very early work on anthrax toxins and immunogens is reviewed by Eurich and Hewlett (1930). Lincoln and Fish (1970) provide two further early references as well as a thorough review of the numerous and extensive developments which took place from World War II to 1967.

The period leading up to and following the 1972 Biological Weapons Convention and the associated demise in the official focus on biological weapons resulted in a decade in which interest in anthrax was almost totally lost. It was a relatively short-lived interlude, however, which was brought to an end by the Sverdlovsk incident in 1979 (Meselson et al. 1994; Guilleman 1999). This, together with the Gulf War in 1991 and the more insidious recent development of new fears about bioterrorism (Henderson 1999; McGovern et al. 1999; Franz and Zajtchuk 2000), in turn produced successive new waves of intense defence-funded research into anthrax which has led to an almost unprecedented leap forward in the understanding of the organism and its pathogenic mechanisms at the molecular-genetic level (Little and Ivins 1999; Turnbull 2000; Turnbull et al. 2000). The stimulus to further research has now been markedly reinforced by the bioterrorist events in the USA involving anthrax in the last quarter of 2001. With the sequences of the virulence plasmids recently revealed (Okinaka et al. 1999) and that of the whole genome nearing completion (Read and Peterson 1999), the long and fascinating history of anthrax, far from coming to an end, is about to receive another significant boost with a host of new revelations and new understanding of its evolution and genealogy and of its ecology and pathogenesis. From this will undoubtedly follow soon associated practical developments in its surveillance, diagnosis, detection and control (including prophylaxis and therapy).

2
Aetiology and Ecology

Anthrax is a bacterial disease caused by the aerobic spore-forming *Bacillus anthracis*, a Gram-positive, rod-shaped bacterium. In keeping with other spore-formers, when conditions are not conducive to growth and multiplication of the bacilli, they form spores. Sporulation of *B. anthracis* requires the presence of free oxygen; within the anaerobic environment of the infected host the organism is in the vegetative form.

Although *B. anthracis* multiplies readily on or in basic laboratory nutrient agars or broths, the vegetative forms appear to be poor survivors in simple environments such as water or milk and more dependent than other *Bacillus* species on sporulation for species survival (Turnbull et al. 1991; Bowen et al. 1992; Lindeque and Turnbull 1994).

Outside the laboratory, multiplication by *B. anthracis* occurs almost invariably within an animal host and the organism is, therefore, essentially an obligate pathogen. The spore forms, on the other hand, are highly resistant to adverse environmental conditions and are, therefore, both the predominant phase in the environment and the centre of the ecological cycle of the organism (Fig. 1).

Within the infected host the spores germinate to produce the vegetative forms that multiply, eventually killing the host. A proportion of the bacilli shed by the dying or dead animal into the environment (usually soil under the carcass) sporulate, ready to be taken up by another animal. The rate of sporulation by the shed vegetative cells and the proportion which succeed in sporulating are influenced in a complex manner by the environmental conditions into which they fall. Temperature, pH, a_w, oxygen availability, sunlight, organic matter and the presence of certain cations such as Mn^{++} are among the many influencing factors.

The extent to which subsidiary cycles of germination, multiplication and resporulation occur in the environment remains a topic of debate, but research (TURNBULL et al. 1991; BOWEN et al. 1992; LINDEQUE and TURNBULL 1994) suggests that the level of nutrient required for this to become possible is unlikely to occur very frequently under natural conditions. Spores can germinate outside an animal if they fall into appropriate conditions, i.e. a temperature between about 8° and 45 °C, a pH between about 5 and 9, a relative humidity greater than 95% and the presence of adequate nutrients, but, as indicated above, the vegetative forms are poor survivors and are likely to die rather than multiply if nutritional conditions or the concentration of protective organic matter are insufficient. Nevertheless, the fact that contamination levels at a carcass site can sometimes remain apparently undiminished for years after the death of the animal despite exposure of the site to wind, rain and sunlight (TURNBULL et al. 1998) is hard to explain in terms other than localized multiplication.

The exceptional degree of monomorphism in this species (see the chapter by P. KEIM and K.L. SMITH, this volume) is attributable to two principal factors. First, because its multiplication cycles depend almost exclusively on infections in animal hosts and, often, considerable time intervals (sometimes decades) separate sequential hosts, the opportunities *B. anthracis* has to multiply are rare compared with other pathogenic species. In the second place, because vegetative forms within the bac-

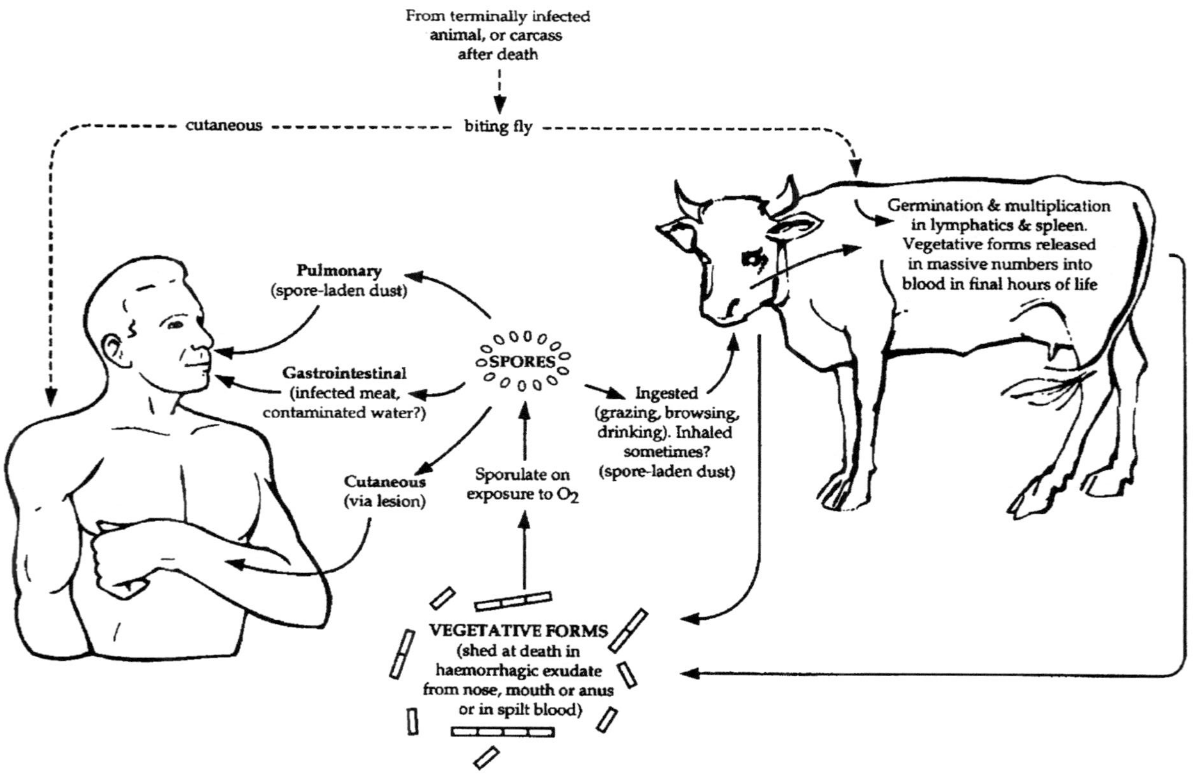

Fig. 1. Cycle of infection in anthrax. The spore is central to the cycle, although infection can also be acquired through uptake of the vegetative forms when, for example, humans or carnivores eat meat from an animal that died of anthrax or when biting flies transmit the disease

terium's life cycle develop almost exclusively within an animal host, they are rarely exposed to the mutagens, phages or other environmental factors which bring about strain variation in other bacterial species.

3 Epidemiology and Transmission

According to reports received by the Office International des Epizooties (OIE), few countries are truly enzootic for anthrax. On the other hand, few escape the occasional case in their livestock. The principal endemic areas in the world today are in sub-Saharan Africa, central and southern Asia and certain regions of China. Haiti is an isolated 'hot spot' and the disease remains well recognised in southern Europe, including Turkey, and the Middle East. Because humans almost invariably contract anthrax from contact, directly or indirectly, with infected animals, an approximate assessment of the extent of the disease in the livestock of those countries where disease monitoring in livestock is very limited can be made from a knowledge of its incidence in the human population. Historical analysis of epidemiological data globally reveals the approximate ratios of 1 human cutaneous anthrax case to 10 anthrax livestock carcasses and 1 incident of enteric human anthrax to 30–60 anthrax-infected animals eaten (Turnbull et al. 1998).

In the past it was epidemiologically convenient to divide human anthrax into non-industrial and industrial, reflecting the relationship between occupation and exposure. Non-industrial anthrax referred to its occurrence in farmers, butchers and veterinarians, whereas the industrial form alludes to its occurrence in persons employed in the processing of bones, hides, wool and other animal products. It is more common nowadays to find anthrax divided in terms of the route by which the disease was acquired, i. e. cutaneous anthrax acquired through a skin lesion, oropharyngeal/gastrointestinal anthrax contracted from ingestion of contaminated food, primarily meat from an animal that died of the disease and inhalational (pulmonary) anthrax from breathing in airborne anthrax spores.

Non-industrial anthrax generally results from handling infected carcasses but also includes the disease as transmitted by insect bites or acquired by ingestion; it usually takes the cutaneous form of the disease, therefore, or occasionally the oropharyngeal/gastrointestinal form, and tends to be seasonal in parallel with the seasonal incidence in the animals from which it is contracted. Industrial anthrax also commonly takes the cutaneous form but has a far higher probability than non-industrial anthrax of taking the inhalational form through intake of spore-laden dust.

Anthrax is a seasonal disease; its incidence in any one place is related in a complex manner to temperature, rains or drought and soil type, which, in turn, also affect population density and host condition. Much is hypothesised but little is proven about the roles, separately or together, of these factors in the incidence of the disease. At the most simplistic level, climate probably acts directly or indirectly by influencing the way in which an animal comes into contact with the spores (for example, grazing closer to the soil in dry periods when grass is short or sparse, or movement of herds to restricted sites when water becomes scarce) and/or by affecting the general state of health of the hosts and, thereby, their level of resistance to infection from the stress which results when meteorological conditions lead to diminished food and water sources, crowding around the remaining sources, heat, high concentrations of insects and hormonal changes heralding the onset of the rutting season.

Despite the disease being so well recognised for so long, it is amazing how little is known about how animals acquire anthrax. It is generally believed that ingestion of the spores while grazing or browsing is the usual route of infection. *B. anthracis* is not an invasive organism and needs a lesion in the skin or mucosa in which to lodge and initiate infection and, for animals taking up the spores while grazing or browsing, it is assumed that grit or spiky leaves, grass, etc. produce these in the oral, pharyngeal or intestinal mucosa. However, such attempts as have been made to understand oral-route infection in animals have usually failed to explain what occurs in the field to any degree of satisfaction. It has generally proved difficult, and to require very large doses (far larger than would ever be expected to be encountered in the field in natural infections), to infect species generally regarded as susceptible to anthrax by the oral route (DRUETT et al. 1953; SHLINGMAN et al. 1956; DE VOS 1990; REDMOND et al. 1997; CARTER and PEARSON 1999). Inhalation of spores while grazing over contaminated sites which are dry and dusty is another possible means of infection (DE VOS and TURNBULL 2001).

Incrimination of insects in transmission of anthrax dates back as far as 1863 (QUINN and TURNBULL 1998) and both biting and non-biting flies were evidently considered in the early 1900s to be important as transmitters of anthrax (Sen and Minett 1944). Spread by biting flies has been used to explain explosive epizootics (Davies 1983) and it has been shown experimentally that anthrax can be transmitted by the bites of insects (Sen and Minett 1944); Turell and Knudson 1987). Non-biting flies have been incriminated as the principal vector of anthrax in browsing herbivores (de Vos 1990).

Both for animals and humans, anthrax transmission is considered to be of the point-source type; direct animal-to-animal transmission of the disease in animals appears to be confined to carnivores consuming anthrax carcasses or, occasionally, osteophagia (licking bones to supply calcium and/or phosphorus in conditions where they are deficient in the diet [Sterne 1959; Ebedes 1976]). However, the occasional occurrence of very large outbreaks, involving hundreds of herbivorous animals, is often hard to explain in terms of point-source infection. It is made harder by the fact that, in such outbreaks, usually one species is affected while other susceptible species with apparently equal opportunity for exposure suffer no losses or only a few. This is particularly readily seen in wildlife epizootics. Arthropod transmission may partly account for epizootics, but again the research that might explain the species specificity of epizootics in terms of arthropod transmission has not been done.

Accounts of person-to-person transmission of anthrax are also extremely rare (Heyworth et al. 1975; Lalitha et al.1988; Quinn and Turnbull 1998). Transmission by biting insects is again believed to be at least an occasional mechanism by which anthrax is contracted by humans (Rao and Mohiyudeen 1958; Davies 1983).

4
Clinical Manifestations

Sudden death in an animal without prior symptoms or after a brief period of fever and disorientation should lead to suspicion of anthrax. Bloody fluid exuding from the nose, mouth or anus of the dead animal is particularly suggestive. In pigs and carnivores, local oedemas, particularly in the neck region, are further suggestive signs. At death in most susceptible species, the blood contains 10^7 to 10^9 bacilli per millilitre provided the animal has not been treated; pigs are an exception and the bacterium is usually present in low numbers or may be undetectable in blood at death.

Of the three forms of the disease in humans, cutaneous, inhalational and alimentary tract anthrax, the cutaneous form accounts for well over 95% of cases on record. In cutaneous anthrax, approximately 3–5 days (range 1–12 days) after entry of the infecting *B. anthracis* through a lesion in the skin, a small pimple or papule appears. Over the next 2–3 days, the centre of the pimple ulcerates to become a dry, black, firmly adherent scab surrounded by a ring of vesicles. This is the characteristic anthrax eschar. Pain is usually minimal and pain and pus generally reflect secondary infection of the lesion. The lesions vary greatly in size from about 2 cm to several centimetres across and are always accompanied by substantial oedema which may extend a long way from the lesion. In the case of lesions on the face or neck, the oedema may endanger life by compressing the trachea and tracheotomy may be necessary. In uncomplicated cases, the eschar begins to resolve about 10 days after the appearance of the initial papule and resolution takes 2–6 weeks, regardless of treatment, usually leaving minor scarring. Historical records before availability of treatment show that less than 20% of untreated cutaneous cases were fatal.

There are two clinical forms of anthrax of the alimentary tract: oropharyngeal anthrax, in which the main clinical features are sore hroat, dysphagia, fever, regional lymphadenopathy in the neck and toxaemia, and intestinal anthrax where symptoms are non-specific and variously include nausea, vomiting, fever, abdominal pain, haematemesis, bloody diarrhoea and ascites generally terminating in the rapid onset of prostration, shock, collapse and death.

The outcome of the bioterrorist events involving anthrax in the USA in the last quarter of 2001 has been thorough descriptions of the clinical details of inhalational anthrax. Analysis of 10 of the cases associated with the bioterrorist events of 2001 (Jernigan et al. 2001) revealed a median incubation period of 4 days (range 4–6 days) and a variety of symptoms at initial presentation, most of the patients exhibiting fever or chills, sweats, fatigue or malaise, minimal or non-productive cough, dyspnea, and nausea or vomiting. All had abnormal chest X-rays, the majority with infiltrates, pleural effusion, and mediastinal widening. Mediastinal lymphadenopathy was present in seven cases. Again, untreated initial mild symptoms end in sudden shock, collapse and death, all occurring within a few hours. Meningitis is a potential complication. Second infections in the same individual are clearly rare but not unheard of (Christie 1969; Heyworth et al. 1975).

5
Pathology

The information available on the pathology of anthrax mostly comes from studies in the 1940s to 1960s (BARNES 1947; YOUNG et al. 1946; ROSS 1955, 1957; WIDDICOMBE et al. 1956; GLEISER 1967; GLEISER et al. 1968; DALLDORF et al. 1971). It was observed then that the nodes act as centres for the proliferation and dissemination of the bacilli leading to septicaemia and death. Cutaneous infection results in oedema, cellular infiltration and multiplication of the bacilli with the regional lymph nodes becoming enlarged, haemorrhagic and containing the bacilli. Inhalation anthrax involves less activity at the site of invasion and changes in lung parenchyma, such as hyperaemia, oedema and cellular infiltration are mild or absent (YOUNG et al. 1946). The bacilli do not multiply in the lung itself but lead to infection of the mediastinal lymph nodes; the alveolar lining acts merely as a point of entry by the bacilli with multiplication and subsequent bacteraemia only occurring after infection of the lymph nodes draining the lungs (BARNES 1947). There was no evidence that inhaled anthrax spores reached the blood stream direct from the lung (ROSS 1957).

The earliest histological changes in the lymph nodes and spleen are necrosis of germinal centres; as infection proceeds, the nodes become oedematous and then haemorrhagic; veins and capillaries within the nodes become filled with thrombi composed of leukocytes, platelets, fibrin and bacteria (DALLDORF et al. 1971). On occasion pneumonia does result from oedema and haemorrhage with thrombosis of the pulmonary vascular bed, though it is not clear whether this represents primary infection or re-infection (DALLDORF et al. 1971). In a comparison of susceptible and resistant species, GLEISER (1967) found marked differences in the response in the lung to aerosol infection. Intense fibrinous and cellular responses found in the resistant species, as compared with mild cellular and fibrinous responses in susceptible animals, was seen as representing an ability to 'wall off' the pathogen by the massive deposits of fibrin and the surrounding activity of the cellular infiltrations.

The basic disease mechanism is vascular injury with oedema, haemorrhage and thrombosis recognised as being the result of action of the toxin on the endothelial cell membranes which rendered them permeable to plasma and caused adhesion of leukocytes and platelets with widespread intravascular thrombosis (Dalldorf et al. 1971). The molecular action of the toxin, and its detailed role in the pathogenesis of anthrax, has been progressively elucidated over the past two decades and is covered in the chapter by D.B. Lacy and R.J. Collier (this volume).

6 Bacteriology

Bacillus anthracis is a Gram-positive, non-motile, aerobic, facultatively anaerobic, spore-forming bacterium. The vegetative form is a square-ended rod, 1 – 1.5 μm by 5 – 8 μm. In infected blood or tissue the rods are present singly and in short chains surrounded by the polypeptide capsule visible under the microscope when stained with polychrome methylene blue (M'Fadyean reaction). In stained smears made from colonies on nutrient agar plates or from broth cultures, the bacteria are seen in endless filaments and there is no capsule unless special conditions are met. For agar cultures, the medium needs to contain bicarbonate (approximately 0.7%) and be incubated under 5%–20% CO_2; liquid cultures need to contain at least 50% serum (horse serum appears to be best).

The characteristic morphology is an immediate aid to identification of a colony as being that of *B. anthracis*. After overnight incubation on blood agar, it is white or grey-white, 2–4 mm in diameter, bee's-eye in texture, non-haemolytic (or very weakly haemolytic), and distinctly tacky; the growth can be made to stand up from the colony with an inoculating loop. This is the result of its growth in long chains. The usual confirmatory tests on a colony meeting this description are lysis by the diagnostic ('gamma') phage, sensitivity to penicillin and production of the capsule during growth in blood or serum or on bicarbonate agar under 5%–20% CO_2. In addition, the toxin and capsule genes can be amplified with the polymerase chain reaction (PCR).

In conventional physiological and biochemical systems for differentiation of *Bacillus* species, only motility, haemolysis and the production of capsule have proved particularly helpful as differential characteristics for separating *B. anthracis* from *B. cereus*. Gordon et al. (1973) list citrate utilisation, decomposition of tyrosine, growth at 45 °C and failure to digest litmus milk as helpful tests but none of these approached 100% reliability. It is probably fair to say that the publication of Gordon et al. (1973) effectively replaced earlier papers in which other differential criteria were put forward (Knight and Proom 1950; Burdon 1956; Burdon and Wende 1960). Other minor differences can be seen in a tabulated profile of *Bacillus* species (Logan and Turnbull 1999). The bottom line, however, is that an isolate with the correct colonial morphology which is non-haemolytic or very weakly haemolytic, non-motile, sensitive to penicillin and the diagnostic ('gamma') phage, and which produces the characteristic capsule of *B. anthracis* under appropriate (but simple) growth conditions is *B. anthracis*. In the last few years, the PCR has become a powerful additional tool with which to demonstrate that the genes for both virulence factors, the capsule and the toxin, are present (Turnbull et al. 1998). Other biochemical and physiological tests contribute virtually nothing to the identification of this bacterium and these screening tests should be done even when utilising any of the several available commercial identification systems if there is any thought that the isolate may be *B. anthracis*.

The dependence on virulence factors for differentiation of *B. anthracis* from its close relatives is well recognised and, until recently, the existence of occasional ambiguous isolates lacking the genes for one or both of the virulence factors, and therefore incapable of causing anthrax, has only mattered to taxonomists. However, strategic and economic considerations have now made it important to a wider community, including defence, health care and agricultural bodies, that unambiguous identification of any suspect isolate which does not fit the criteria listed above in an absolute manner should be possible (Turnbull 1999). Considerable research effort has been targeted at this goal in the last 3–5 years and, as indicated at the outset of this chapter, the newly emerging *B. anthracis* genome sequence can be expected to contribute greatly to this ongoing effort (Turnbull et al. 2000).

References

Anon (1918) Report of the departmental committee appointed to inquire as to precautions for preventing danger of infection from anthrax in the manipulation of wool, goat hair, and camel hair. Vol. II. Report of the Committee, p. 13. HMSO, London

Barnes JM (1947) The development of anthrax following the administration of spores by inhalation. Br J Exp Pathol 28:385–394

Bowen JE, Turnbull PCB (1992) The fate of *Bacillus anthracis* in unpasteurized and pasteurized milk. Lett Appl Microbiol 15:224–227

Brachmann PS (1991) In: Evans ES, Brachmann PS (eds) Bacterial infections of humans. Epidemiology and control, 2nd edn. Plenum Medical Book Co, New York, pp 75–86

Burdon KL (1956) Useful criteria for the identification of *Bacillus anthracis* and related species. J Bacteriol 71:25–42

Burdon KL, Wende RD (1960) On the differentiation of anthrax bacilli from *Bacillus cereus*. J Infect Dis 107:224–234

Carter GB (1992) Porton Down. 75 years of chemical and biological research. HMSO, London

Carter G, Balmer B (1999) Chemical and biological warfare and defence, 1945–90. In: Bud R, Gummett P (eds) Cold war, hot science. Applied research in Britain's defence laboratories, 1945–1990. Harwood Academic Publishers, Australia, Canada, The Netherlands

Carter GB, Pearson GS (1999) British biological warfare and biological defence, 1925–45. In: Geissler E, van Courtland Moon JE (eds) Biological and toxin weapons: research, development and use from the Middle Ages to 1945. Oxford University Press, pp 168–189

Choquette LPE, Broughton E (1981) In: Davis JW, Karsted LH, Trainer DO (eds) Infectious diseases of wild mammals, 2nd edn. Iowa State University Press, Ames, Iowa, pp 288–296

Christie AB (1969) Infectious Diseases: Epidemiology and Clinical Practice. E&S Livingstone Ltd, Edinburgh, pp 752–779

Christie AB (1987) Anthrax. In: Christie AB (ed) Infectious diseases: epidemiology and clinical practice, 4th edn. Churchill Livingstone, London, pp 983–1003

Cole SW (1847) The American veterinarian or diseases of domestic animals. John P. Jewett & Co., Boston, pp 214–217

Dalldorf FG, Kaufmann AF, Brachman PS (1971) Woolsorter's disease. Arch Pathol 92:418–426

De Vos V (1990) The ecology of anthrax in the Kruger National Park, South Africa. Salisbury Med Bull No 68 (special suppl), 19–23

De Vos V, Turnbull PCB (2001) Anthrax. In: Coetzer CAWJ, Thompson GR, Tustin RC, Kriek NNPJ (eds) Infectious diseases of livestock, with special reference to South Africa, 2nd edn. Oxford University Press, Cape Town (in press)

Dirckx, JM (1981). Virgil on anthrax. Am J Dermatopathol 3:191–195

Davies JCA (1983) A major epidemic of anthrax in Zimbabwe. Central Afr J Med 29:8–12

Druett HA, Henderson DW, Packman L, Peacock S (1953) Studies on respiratory infection with anthrax spores. I. The influence of particle size on respiratory infection with anthrax spores. J Hyg 51:359–371

Ebedes H (1976) Anthrax epizootics in Etosha National Park. Madoqua 10:99–118

Eurich FW, Hewlett RT (1930) *Bacillus anthracis*. In: A system of bacteriology in relation to medicine. HMSO, London, pp 439–478

Franz DR, Zajtchuk R (2000) Biological terrorism: understanding the threat, preparation, and medical response. Disease-a-Month 46:129–190

Geissler E (1999) Biological warfare activities in Germany, 1923–45. In: Geissler E, van Courtland Moon JE (eds) Biological and toxin weapons: research, development and use from the Middle Ages to 1945. Oxford University Press, pp 91–126

GLASSMAN HN (1966) Discussion (industrial inhalation anthrax). Bacteriol Rev 30:657–659

GLEISER CA (1967) Pathology of anthrax infection in animal hosts. Fed Proc 26: 1518–1521

GLEISER CA, GOCHENOUR WS, WARD MK (1968) Pulmonary lesions in dogs and pigs exposed to a cloud of anthrax spores. J Comp Pathol 78:445–449

GORDON RE, HAYNES WC, PANG CH-N (1973) The Genus Bacillus. Agricultural Research Service, Agriculture Handbook No. 427. Washington DC, USDA

GUILLEMIN J (1999) Anthrax. The Investigation of a Deadly Outbreak. University of California Press, Berkeley and Los Angeles, p 321

HAMBLETON P, CARMAN JA, MELING J (1984) Anthrax: The disease in relation to vaccines. Vaccine 2:125–132

HANNA PC, ACOSTA D, COLLIER RJ (1993) On the role of macrophages in anthrax. Proc Natl Acad Sci USA 90:10198–10201

HENDERSON DA (1999) The looming threat of bioterrorism. Science 283:1279–1282

HEYWORTH B, ROPP ME, VOOS UG, MEINEL HI, DARLOW HM (1975) Anthrax in the Gambia: an epidemiological study. Brit Med J 4:79–82

HUTYRA F, MAREK J (1922) Special Pathology and Therapeutics of the Diseases of Domestic Animals, 2nd American edn, Baillière, Tindall and Cox, Chicago and London

JERNIGAN JA, STEPHENS DS, ASHFORD DA, OMENACA C, TOPIEL MS, GALBRAITH M, TAPPER M, FISK TL, ZAKI S, POPOVIC T, MEYER RF, QUINN CP, HARPER SA, FRIDKIN SK, SEJVAR JJ, SHEPARD CW, MCCONNELL M, GUARNER J, SHIEH W-J, MALECKI JM, GERBERDING JL, HUGHES JM, PERKINS BA (2001) Bioterrorism-related inhalational anthrax: the first 10 cases reported in the United States. Emerg Infect Dis 7:933–944. *This article is available from website www.bt.cdc.gov in downloadable format*

KLEMM DM, KLEMM WR (1959) A history of anthrax. J Am Vet Med Assoc 135: 458–462

KNIGHT BCJG, PROOM H (1950) A comparative survey of the nutrition and physiology of mesophilic species in the genus *Bacillus*. J Gen Microbiol 4:508–538

LALITHA MK, ANANDI V, WALTER N, DEVADATTA JO, PULIMOOD BM (1988) Primary anthrax presenting as an injection abscess. Ind J Pathol Microbiol 31:254–256

LINCOLN RE, FISH DC (1970) Anthrax toxin. In: Montie TC, Kadis S, Ajl SJ (eds) Microbial Toxins III. Academic Press, New York, pp 361–414

LITTLE SF, IVINS BE (1999) Molecular pathogenesis of *Bacillus anthracis* infection. Microbes Infect 2:131–139

LITTLE SF, LEPPLA SH, BURNETT JW, FRIEDLANDER AMF (1994) Structure-function analysis of *Bacillus anthracis* edema factor by using monoclonal antibodies. Biochem Biophys Res Commun 199:676–682

LOGAN NA, TURNBULL PCB (1999) *Bacillus* and recently derived genera. In: Murray PR, Baron EJ, Pfaller MA, Tenover FC, Yolken RH (eds) Manual of clinical microbiology, 6th edn. ASM Press, Washington DC, pp 357–369

MCGOVERN TW, CHRISTOPHER GW, EITZEN EM (1999) Cutaneous manifestations of biological warfare and related threat agents. Arch Dermatol 135:311–322

Meselson M, Guillemin J, Hugh-Jones M, Langmuir A, Popova I, Shelokov A, Ampolskaya O (1994) The Sverdlovsk anthrax outbreak of 1979. Science 266: 1202–1208

Okinaka R, Cloud K, Hampton O, Hoffmaster AR, Hill KK, Keim P, Koehler TM, Lamke G, Mahillon J, Manter D, Martinez Y, Ricke D, Svensson R, Jackson PJ (1999) Sequence and organization of pXO1, the large *Bacillus anthracis* plasmid harboring the anthrax toxin genes. J. Bacteriol 181:6509–6515

Parvizpour D (1978) Human anthrax in Iran. An epidemiological study of 468 cases. Intl J Zoon 5:69–74

Plotkin SA, Brachman PS, Utell M, Bumford FH, Atchison MM (1960) An epidemic of inhalation anthrax, the first in the twentieth century. Am J Med 29:992–1001

Quinn CP, Turnbull PCB (1998) Anthrax. In: Collier L, Balows A, Sussman M (eds), Topley & Wilson's Microbiology and Microbial Infections, 9th edn, vol 3. Arnold, London, pp 799–818

Rao KNS, Mohiyudeen S (1958) Tabanus flies as transmitters of anthrax – a field experience. Indian Vet J 35:348–353

Read T, Peterson S (1999) Whole genome sequencing of *Bacillus anthracis.* Abstracts of the 2nd International Workshop on the molecular biology of *Bacillus cereus, Bacillus anthracis* and *Bacillus thuringiensis.* Taos, New Mexico, August 11–13, 1999

Redmond C, Hall GA, Turnbull PCB, Gillgan JS (1997) Experimentally assessed public health risks associated with pigs from farms experiencing anthrax. Vet Rec 141:244–247

Redmond C, Pearce MJ, Manchee RJ, Berdal BP (1998) Deadly relic of the Great War. Nature 393:747–748

Ross JM (1955) On the histopathology of experimental anthrax in the guinea-pig. Br J Exp Pathol 36:336–339

Ross JM (1957) The pathogenesis of anthrax following the administration of spores by the respiratory route. J Pathol Bacteriol 73:485–494

Salmon DE (1896) Anthrax. In: Special report on diseases of the horse. Government Printing Office, Washington, pp 526–530

Schlingman AS, Devlin HB, Wright GG, Maine RJ, Manning M (1956) Immunizing activity of alum-precipitated protective antigen of *Bacillus anthracis* in cattle, sheep and swine. Am J Vet Res 17:256–261

Sen SK, Minett FC (1944) Experiments on the transmission of anthrax through flies. Indian J Vet Sci Ani Husb 14:149–158

Smith KL, deVos V, Bryden H, Hugh-Jones ME, Keim P, Price LB, Klevytska A, Scholl DT (1999) Meso-scale ecology of anthrax in southern Africa: a pilot study of diversity and clustering. J Appl Microbiol 87:204–207

Sterne M (1937) The effects of different carbon dioxide concentrations on the growth of virulent anthrax strains. Pathogenicity and immunity tests on guinea pigs and sheep with anthrax variants derived from virulent strains. Ond J Vet Sci An Ind 9:49–67

Sterne M (1959) Anthrax. In: Stableforth AW, Galloway IA (eds) Infectious Diseases of Animals. Diseases due to Bacteria, vol. I. Butterworths Scientific Publications, London, pp 16–52

Sterne M (1967) Distribution and economic importance of anthrax. Fed Proc 26:1493–1495

Turell MJ, Knudson GB (1987) Mechanical transmission of *Bacillus anthracis* by stable flies (*Stomoxys calcitrans*) and mosquitoes (*Aedes aegypti* and *Aedes taeniorhynchus*). Infect Immun 55:1859–1861

Turnbull PCB (1998) Anthrax. In: Palmer SR, Soulsby L, Simpson D (eds) Textbook of Zoonoses Control, Oxford University Press, 3–16

Turnbull PCB (1999) Definitive identification of *Bacillus anthracis* – a review. J Appl Microbiol 87:237–240

Turnbull PCB (2000) Current status of immunization against anthrax: old vaccines may be here to stay for a while. Curr Opin Infect Dis 13:113–120

Turnbull PCB, Quinn CP, Henderson I (2001) *Bacillus anthracis* and other *Bacillus* species. In: Sussman M (ed) Molecular Medical Microbiology, Academic Press, London, pp 2011–2031

Turnbull PCB, Bell RHV, Saigawa K, Munyenyembe FEC, Mulenga CK, Makala LHC (1991) Anthrax in wildlife in the Luangwa Valley, Zambia. Vet Rec 128:399–403

Turnbull PCB, Böhm R, Cosivi O, Doganay M, Hugh-Jones ME, Joshi DD, Lalitha MK, de Vos V (1998) Guidelines on surveillance and control of anthrax in humans and animals. WHO/EMC/ZDI/98.6

Turnbull PCB, Jackson PJ, Hill KK, Keim P, Kolstø A-B, Beecher DJ (2000) Longstanding taxonomic enigmas within the '*Bacillus cereus* group' are on the verge of being resolved by far-reaching molecular developments. Forecasts on the possible outcome by an *ad hoc* team. In: Berkeley RCW, Logan NA, Heyndrickx M, de Vos P (eds) Applications and systematics of *Bacillus* and relatives. Blackwell Science Ltd, Oxford

Turnbull PCB, Lindeque PM, Le Roux J, Bennett AM, Parks SR (1998) Airborne movement of anthrax spores from carcass sites in the Etosha National Park, Namibia. J Appl Microbiol 84:667–676

Wheelis M (1999) Biological sabotage in World War I. In: Geissler E, van Courtland Moon JE (eds) Biological and toxin weapons: research, development and use from the Middle Ages to 1945. Oxford University Press, pp 35–69

Widdicombe JG, Hughes R, May AJ (1956) The role of the lymphatic system in the pathogenesis of anthrax. Br J Exp Pathol 37:343–349

Wilson GS, Miles A (1946) Anthrax. In: Topley and Wilson's principles of bacteriology, virology and immunity, 3rd edn. Edward Arnold, London, pp 1730–1745

Young GA, Zelle MR, Lincoln RE (1946) Respiratory pathogenicity of *Bacillus anthracis* spores. 1. Methods of study and observations on pathogenesis. J Infect Dis 79:233–245

CHAPTER 2

Bacillus anthracis Evolution and Epidemiology

P. KEIM, K. L. SMITH

Abstract. *Bacillus anthracis* is a pathogen that is widely distributed around the globe. However, this great distribution is not accompanied by great genetic diversity. Although subtle morphological and biochemical differences exist, the underlying genetic basis for this plasticity is not known. Indeed, very few single nucleotide differences have been detected among isolates and the only documented high variable sequences are associated with variable number tandem repeated (VNTR) sequences. The differences among the VNTRs has been used to suggest phylogenetic relationships among the worldwide isolates. There is one major clonal split in *B. anthracis* (A and B), with two minor clusters established within the B branch and four or more minor branches within the A group. The A branch is the most common worldwide, though the B branch is locally important in certain areas. The ecology and the evolution of *B. anthracis* have been greatly influenced by the spore phase of the lifecycle.

P. KEIM, K. L. SMITH
Department of Biological Sciences, Northern Arizona University, Flagstaff, AZ 86011-5640, USA, Email: Paul.Keim@nau.edu.

1 Taxonomic Considerations

Traditional systematics have sought to group individuals into divisions based on common features. At some level, this aggregation ignores or minimizes differences among individuals to make these taxonomic groups. *Bacillus anthracis* was a relatively straightforward species designation based on the ability of bacterial isolates to cause the easily identified disease of anthrax. In practice, this involved isolation of the pathogen from anthrax victims. This clear traditional criterion was aided in this case by limited differences among isolates. *Bacillus anthracis* appears to be one of the most homogeneous bacterial species described because of: (1) the traditionally very narrow taxonomic definition (Helgason et al. 2000); (2) slow evolutionary progression; and (3) probably a recent common ancestor to all known isolates.

Indeed, the great homogeneity is in part artificial and a function of how systematics has been applied to this pathogen. Helgason et al. (2000) argue that *B. anthracis* is undeserving of the species-level designation, being merely a clonal lineage of *B. cereus*. Using both multiple enzyme electrophoresis (MEE) and multiple locus sequence typing (MLST), *B. anthracis* strains are associated with particular *B. cereus* strains. Some of these are pathogenic, whereas others are not. A periodontitis strain is certainly one of the closest non-anthrax-causing relatives on the basis of both MEE and MLST. But other close relatives are nonpathogenic and even considered beneficial. The most obvious difference between these isolates is the presence of virulence plasmids, but chromosome-based differences may be present as well. The great similarity in gene sequences among these strains argues for a recent common ancestor but does not preclude whole gene differences. Horizontal transfer via plasmids has obviously occurred, and chromosomal gene transfer or loss could have occurred also. The genetic composition of these similar isolates leads to their very unique biological properties.

2 Phenotypic Variation Among Strains

Variation among *B. anthracis* isolates is rare and somewhat confusing perhaps because it does not always have a genetic basis. Although there is not enough phenotypic variation for detailed differentiation among natural isolates, the variation that has been seen illustrates that this is not strictly a monotypic species.

Early reports (1900 to about 1960) on phenotypic variation deal mainly with the plasticity of *B. anthracis* colony morphology and because of a lack of understanding of capsule formation culture requirements (STERNE 1937a, b, 1938). This literature describes rough, smooth, phantom, and mucoid colony types. It has since been discovered that capsule formation in culture is differentially controlled by temperature and CO_2 concentrations (EZZELL and WELKOS 1999). Observations of physiological parameters were complicated by the affect of pXO2 plasmid loss on capsule formation, which, of course, is a phenomenon with a real genetic basis.

As better control over culture conditions have been developed, subtler differences in colony attributes have become detectable. *B. anthracis* is generally described as having gray to white colonies on agar with a ground glass appearance, tenacious, and butyrous. But this is variable, and the variation seems to be related to genetic affiliations. SMITH et al. (2000) noted genotypic group associations related to colony morphology while working with a worldwide collection of *B. anthracis* isolates. "A" type isolates (see below) are consistently less tenacious than "B" type isolates. B isolates are emulsified in buffered solutions with difficulty and even appear slimy. Tenacity of particular strains can be demonstrated by drawing a bacteriological loop across *B. anthracis* colonies grown on agar to form "strings" and give a "tacky" appearance similar to that of drying glue. Such strings may be made to stand perpendicular to the surface of the agar without support. This in vitro variation may be important in the anthrax pathology, as there is a reported association between virulence and tenacity (PARRY et al. 1983). In addition, the association between tenacity and virulence is supported by ecological analysis of anthrax in the Kruger National Park, South Africa. Here, the animal mortality rate is 13 times greater in areas where the Kruger B strains are found compared with areas where Kruger A strains are located. It has been suggested that these differences in tenacity may be a function of chain length attained during growth, although how this would relate to increased virulence is unclear. The genetic basis for this difference is unknown and in need of further investigation.

Variation in growth and sporulation characteristics has been associated with different isolates. In this case, it involves differences between two A-type isolates that are closely related genotypically and both are endemic to Canada. Genotypes (GT) 3 and 5 (KEIM et al. 2000) occur with very little geographic and host overlap. GT 3 occurs in Alberta in cattle, and GT5 occurs further north in wood bison located at the Wood Buffalo Park, Northwest Territories. Yet, in repeated growth and sporulation rate trials under carefully controlled growth conditions, GT5 had significantly higher growth and sporulation rates than GT3 (K. L. Smith and M. Hugh-Jones, unpublished data). This in vitro variation between two isolates could have a role in anthrax pathology. Perhaps the GT 3 adaptation would be to a colder climate, where carcasses cool faster and time after death for maximal growth and sporulation is limited. Likewise, it could be adaptive change to continually proliferating in a host with considerably larger body mass (wood bison vs. domestic cattle). The genetic basis for this variation has not been demonstrated and is in need of further study.

Three traditional and widely diagnostic tests for *B. anthracis* have been gamma phage lysis, lack of motility, and susceptibility to penicillin (Turnbull 1998). But, even with these traits there are reports of *B. anthracis* strains that differ. Early phage selectivity was mitigated by the use of the gamma phage variant, which provided consistent lysis across many *B. anthracis* isolates accounting for its widespread use as a diagnostic tool. However, as larger and more diverse numbers of isolates have been tested, even the gamma phage assay has encountered a few isolates that are phage resistant. Resistance to the gamma phage is undoubtedly caused by a genetic difference, but any association of resistance with genotypic groups and the genes involved is unknown. Similar to gamma phage resistance reports, there are reports of *B. anthracis* isolates displaying motility. Lack of motility has long been considered a diagnostic trait to differentiate *B. anthracis* from other group I bacilli. Most recently there is a report (Liang and Yu 1999) that includes electron micrographs clearly depicting flagella. Hence, the lack of motility is not 100% diagnostic. Finally, penicillin sensitivity has been used as a readily applied diagnostic trait for identification of *B. anthracis*. However, the β-lactamase structural genes are present in the *B. anthracis* genome (P. Keim, unpublished data) and apparently not expressed. Penicillin-resistant mutants are readily selected from wild-type cultures (Pomerantsev et al. 1993), and natural isolates are observed in clinical environments (Lalitha and Thomas 1997). Although *B. anthracis* is a very monomorphic bacterial species, no single diagnostic trait appears to be consistent in all isolates.

3
The *B. anthracis* Genome

The *B. anthracis* genome, of greater than 5 megabasepairs (Mbp), is comprised of the chromosome and two plasmids. Although the sequence of the chromosome is only partially completed at this time, the plasmid sequences have been determined and placed in public databases. The presence of both plasmids is essential for full virulence and really defines an isolate as the anthrax-causing organism. The presence of the plasmids is not sufficient to create virulence, as a few strains have been observed that contain the plasmids but are not virulent. Undoubtedly, there are chromosomal differences between *B. anthracis* and its nearest *Bacilli* relatives, but this will be more subtle than the combined ca. 278 kbp of genetic material contained on the virulence plasmids.

The *B. anthracis* chromosome is presumably a circular DNA molecule with a predicted size of 5–6 mega nucleotide bases. The chromosomal sequencing is being performed by T. Read and colleagues at The Institute for Genome Research (TIGR). Even before completion, the genomic sequence is providing new insights into *B. anthracis* biology. There are ca. 6,700 genes currently predicted by open reading frame (ORF) analysis. About 4,470 of these ORFs have functional assignments based on homology to known genes. The remaining 2,324 ORFs do not have database matches. Approximately 3,250 of the *B. anthracis* ORFs have orthologs identified in the *B. subtilis* genomic sequence. This leaves a large number of genes without orthologs in *B. subtilis* genome and, obviously, a lot of genetics to resolve in *B. anthracis* and its closer relatives. A genome sequencing project (Integrated Genomics) is in progress on a *B. cereus* strain that will help to identify those unique to type I bacilli and those unique to *B. anthracis*. Whether there are significant genetic differences among *B. anthracis* strains is still unresolved, although there are genetic marker differences (see below) and plasmid transfer studies suggest chromosome-based virulence modulators (Ivins et al. 1998).

The toxin gene carrying virulence plasmid (pXO1) has been sequenced from the Sterne strain (Okinaka et al. 1999). It is circular and 181,654 nucleotides in size with 143 ORFs. Sixty-one percent of the DNA is found within predicted ORFs. This plasmid is noted for its toxin genes, *pagA*, *cya*, and *lef*, that have been directly implicated in anthrax pathology (see the chapter by T.M. Koehler, this volume, for more details on these genes). These three genes are located in a 44.8-kbp region flanked by inverted

IS*1627* elements, which has been termed a "pathogenicity island." The inverted repeat structure strongly suggests that the pathogenicity island transposed into the pXO1 plasmid. The inversion of this region has been observed once in laboratory strains (Thorne 1993), demonstrating its potential mobility. On the basis of similarity to known genes, there are 15 putative genes on pXO1 that are implicated in horizontal transfer, including topoisomerases, integrases, and resolvases. Three clustered ORFs are similar to genes from virulent group A *Streptococci* that are involved in synthesis of the serotype-specific polysaccharide capsule. The role of these newly identified genes in the biology of *B. anthracis* is unknown but will be the subject for future studies.

The second virulence plasmid (pXO2) is circular and known to carry three genes (*capBCA*) essential for the biosynthesis of the poly-D-glutamic acid capsule (Ezzell and Welkos 1999). This capsule is unique in its composition but plays a role similar that of to carbohydrate-based capsules as a protective antiphagocytic mechanism. Recently, R. Okinaka and colleagues at Los Alamos National Laboratory determined the sequence of pXO2 from the Pasteur strain. It is 96,231 bp in size with 85 predicted genes (ORFs) and is publicly available from Genbank (accession no. AF188935; http://www.ncbi.nlm.nih.gov:80/entrez). Although the total ORFs identified is 85, 16 of these are small and would encode proteins of less than 100 amino acids. BLAST surveys showed that 69% (59) of the ORFs encode proteins of unknown functions. Putative functions could therefore only be assigned to 26 ORFs on the basis of sequence similarity to proteins found in open databases.

4
Nucleotide Variation Within *B. anthracis*

Single nucleotide polymorphism (SNP) diversity is very low among global isolates of *B. anthracis*. Comparative studies have been performed on the 5′ *vrrB* region of the chromosome and *pagA* gene from pXO1. No nucleotide differences were found in a set of eight very diverse strains in the *vrrB* 5′ coding region and the 5′ noncoding region (Schupp et al. 2000). The total region examined was ca. 800 nucleotides and suggests that the intrinsic diversity value is less than 0.125% per nucleotide. A more comprehensive study of the *pagA* gene on pXO1 involved ca. 2,500 nucleotides in 30 diverse strains (Price et al. 1999). This study provides a better estimate of the intrinsic diversity of the *B. anthracis* genome, and the six polymorphic sites observed translate into a 0.21% diversity per nucleotide. There are not enough data to conclude whether these two estimates are significantly different and whether the observed differences are due to their genomic locations on the chromosome and the pXO1 plasmid. Likewise, there are no studies on pXO2 SNP diversity. The *pagA* SNP data have been used for phylogenetic reconstructions, and these are congruent with other methods primarily based on chromosomal variation (Price et al. 1999; see below). This congruence is inconsistent with plasmid horizontal transfer among the strains studied. Although many technologies are becoming routine for rapid detection and monitoring of SNPs, their low frequency and dispersed genomic locations in *B. anthracis* may be a barrier to their wide application to strain discrimination.

5
Variable Number Tandem Repeats

The first useful molecular variation for strain typing was detected by random genomic sample approaches. Both AP-PCR (arbitrarily primed) and AFLP (amplified fragment length polymorphisms) marker systems interrogate the genome at many dispersed locations. The greatest advantage of these approaches is their universality. No prior sequence data are needed to apply these techniques to a previously unstudied species. In the initial studies among *B. anthracis* strains, AP-PCR (Henderson et al. 1994) detected one polymorphic fragment whereas AFLPs detected 31 polymorphic sites (Keim et al. 1997). These data were used for phylogenetic reconstructions and resulted in the first description of the distinct B types and subdivisions within the A types (Keim et al. 1997). However, one limitation of this type of data is its mostly biallelic nature. Variation is most commonly observed as an amplified PCR fragment present in some strains and not others. When multiple alleles are present, their identification is problematic because of the amplification of many other nonhomologous PCR fragments. In addition, the molecular basis of the variation is usually obscure and can be due to either SNP or structural (e.g., insertion/deletion) changes. Phylogenetic analyses can use molecular mechanistic assumptions to enhance hypothesis formation, but not if the molecular basis of the variation is unknown.

It is now known that both AP-PCR and AFLP variation among *B. anthracis* isolates are primarily based on insertion/deletion differences. Andersen et al. (Andersen et al. 1996) and, subsequently, Jackson et al.

(Jackson et al. 1997) characterized the apparent variation detected by AP-PCR and found a variable number tandem repeated sequence. Variation at this locus (*vrrA*) is due to differing numbers of a 12-bp sequence. It is contained within an ORF, which is undisrupted by the in-frame variation in the repeated sequence. Likewise, AFLP variation has proven largely due to VNTR loci (Keim et al. 1999). About half of the observed AFLP differences among strains are due to length variation, and at least two allelic AFLP fragments are observed. Details of the AFLP variation have been determined for several loci and shown to be due to VNTRs contained within AFLP fragments (Schupp et al. 2000). These have been converted into locus-specific PCR markers, which detect multiple alleles (Keim et al. 2000). However, this random survey approach to identifying VNTRs is tedious and may require months for the development of a single locus marker.

The availability of whole genomic sequences has dramatically changed the detection of molecular diversity. With the use of an informatics approach, over 800 potential VNTRs have been identified on both the chromosome and the plasmids (G. Zinser and P. Keim, unpublished data).

6 *B. anthracis* Evolution

In the absence of sufficient SNPs, molecular variation in VNTRs can be used to identify similarity among *B. anthracis* isolates and to construct phylogenetic hypotheses. An eight-locus VNTR analysis (multiple locus VNTR analysis – MLVA) identified only 89 unique genotypes from over 400 isolates (Keim et al. 2000). There appear to be two major phylogenetic groups or major clonal lineages in this worldwide collection. These were identical to the two major groups identified with AFLPs, which have been labeled as "A" and "B" types (Fig. 1). The "B" lineage accounts for only ~11% of all known strains and is restricted in distribution primarily to southern Africa. Its co-occurrence in this region with members of the genetically distinct A lineage (Smith et al. 1999) has led to speculation that Africa is the origin of *B. anthracis* (Keim et al. 1997). In contrast to B types, isolates from the A lineage are found throughout the world. This contrasting success may be due to stochastic historical dispersal processes or related unique biological features (see below). Minor branching is observed among A types, and about four different subgroups can be recognized (Keim et al. 2000). Some of these groups have biased geographic distribu-

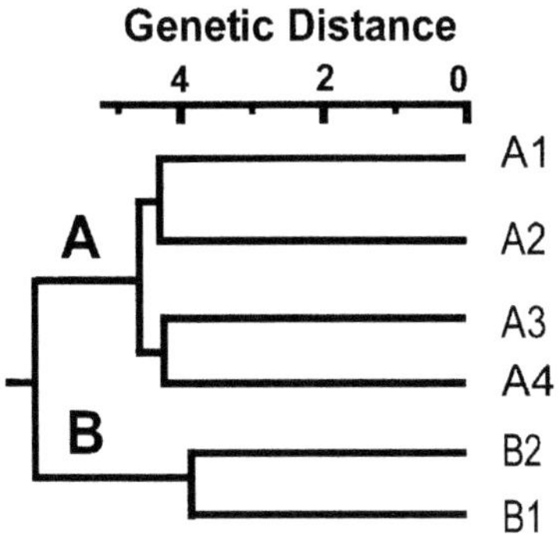

Fig. 1. A phylogenetic model based on VNTR alleles. Similarity among the 89 unique *B. anthracis* MLVA genotypes can be collapsed into six major clonal lineages (after KEIM et al. 2000). The major split is represented by the *A* and *B types*, whereas major subdivisions within each are labeled with *numbers*

tions but are rarely found exclusively in single locations. For example, the A1 group contains the North American endemic group but is also found around the world. The Russian STI vaccine strain is closely related to the North American endemic strains and suggests an Asian/European origin for this group. A large cluster of strains, called the Sterne-Ames group after two well-known members, is responsible for many anthrax outbreaks and is transglobal in distribution. This group may have been spread by human commerce to achieve its wide distribution. In contrast to the wide distribution of major groups, particular genotypes can be found in exclusive locations. Presumably, mutations have occurred during or after distribution that make genotypes at particular locations unique and identifiable.

7 Localized Diversity

The ability to discriminate among *B. anthracis* isolates with MLVA has revealed three general patterns for genetic variation in geographic regions. These patterns are related to the epidemiological origin of the isolates and the history of anthrax in each location.

In a sudden single-source outbreak the diversity is expected to be low or nonexistent. In the north-central Victoria, Australia anthrax outbreak of 1997, 202 cattle and 4 sheep died in a less than 2 months (TURNER et al. 1999a; TURNER et al. 1999b). MLVA showed 28 isolates to be identical

(P. Keim, K. L. Smith and M. Hugh-Jones, unpublished data). All of these isolates must share a recent common ancestor, and this suggests that this outbreak had a single emanating focus. If there was more than one infective foci in this outbreak, those foci must have been derived from a recent common ancestor.

If an endemic strain has enough time, isolates will begin to differentiate because of spontaneous mutations. This appears to be the case in the North American endemic types found in cluster A1 (KEIM et al. 2000). Single marker alleles separate many of the isolates from Canada and the United States and probably represent mutations that have occurred while anthrax has been present in this geographic region. As mentioned above, GT3 occurs in Alberta whereas GT5 occurs further north in the Northwest Territories. In particular, the highly diverse markers on pXO1 and pXO2 differ among North American endemic isolates. These may be the fastest-evolving regions known from the *B. anthracis* genome. Because there is a strong geographic correlation among these isolate subtypes, this suggests distance-dependent dispersal of the pathogen. As *B. anthracis* spreads, it mutates at a slow rate, allowing the epidemiological reconstruct of dispersal routes. If dispersal is slow enough and progressive, the diversity patterns can be very informative on a subcontinental scale.

Finally, there are several examples of very different *B. anthracis* types coexisting in a single geographic area. The best-studied case is from the Kruger National Park, South Africa, where the two of most different isolates known (Kruger A and Kruger B) are found in very close proximity. Indeed, it is this example of differentiation that has led to the suggestion that Africa is the origin of anthrax (KEIM et al. 1997). Although it is possible that Kruger A and B have differentiated locally, it seems more probable that one or both differentiated in other locations and were dispersed to this common site (K. L. Smith et al. unpublished data). Ecological analysis indicates that each strain occupies a unique environmental niche related to soil composition (primarily calcium and pH). This may create a dynamic balancing relationship such that one strain does not dominate the other. Hence, maintenance of the two strains in one location over long time periods requires unique biological properties, but the initial occurrence only needs dispersal. In eastern North America, worldwide importation of contaminated animal products has resulted in many diverse *B. anthracis* isolates. Outbreaks tend to be isolated, and rare occurrences are not due to a single endemic strain or event (M. Hugh-Jones, personal communication). Dispersal over great distances in a short period of time can result in the co-occurrence of greatly differing types. Human commerce seems like the only possible mechanism for such long-range dispersal.

B. anthracis diversity analysis in the Kruger National Park suggests that outbreaks emanate from multiple foci (K.L. Smith et al., unpublished data). A classic view of disease initiation and progression involves a single source with transmission from host to host. Genotypic data coupled with temporal and spatial analysis clearly show coordination among different strain types. Environmental determinants such as temperature, host susceptibility, or rainfall and topology seem to be cuing multiple foci to erupt in a coordinated fashion. This creates a larger outbreak that superficially seems to be emanating from a single focus. The relative weak transmissibility (Turnbull 1998) of *B. anthracis* also argues for multiple but cued outbreaks. Multiple-foci outbreaks may be occurring even if the isolates are identical because of a recent common ancestor. If we think of transmission and outbreaks as long-term temporal events that span decades, anthrax begins to approximate more traditional contagious disease model concepts. Individual outbreaks must be viewed in this context to understand the nature of anthrax epidemiology.

References

Andersen GL, Simchock JM, Wilson KH (1996) Identification of a region of genetic variability among *Bacillus anthracis* strains and related species. J Bacteriol 178: 377–384

Ezzell JW, Welkos SL (1999) The capsule of *Bacillus anthracis,* a review. J Appl Microbiol 87:250

Helgason E et al. (2000) *Bacillus anthracis, Bacillus cereus,* and *Bacillus thuringiensis* – One species on the basis of genetic evidence. Appl Environ Microbiol 66:2627–2630

Henderson I, Duggleby CJ, Turnbull PC (1994) Differentiation of *Bacillus anthracis* from other *Bacillus cereus* group bacteria with the PCR. Int J Syst Bacteriol 44:99–105

Ivins BE et al. (1998) Comparative efficacy of experimental anthrax vaccine candidates against inhalation anthrax in rhesus macaques. Vaccine 16:1141–1148

Jackson PJ et al. (1997) Characterization of the variable-number tandem repeats in vrrA from different *Bacillus anthracis* isolates. Appl Environ Microbiol 63:1400–1405

Keim P et al. (1997) Molecular evolution and diversity in *Bacillus anthracis* as detected by amplified fragment length polymorphism markers. J Bacteriol 179:818–824

Keim P et al. (1999) Molecular diversity in *Bacillus anthracis.* J Appl Microbiol 87: 215–217

Keim P et al. (2000) Multiple-locus variable-number tandem repeat analysis reveals genetic relationships within *Bacillus anthracis.* Journal of Bacteriology 182

Lalitha MK, Thomas MK (1997) Penicillin resistance in *Bacillus anthracis* [letter]. Lancet 349:1522

Liang X, Yu D (1999) Identification of *Bacillus anthracis* strains in China. J Appl Microbiol 87:200–203

Okinaka RT et al. (1999) Sequence and organization of pXO1, the large *Bacillus anthracis* plasmid harboring the anthrax toxin genes. J Bacteriol 181:6509–6515

Parry J, Turnbull P, Gibson R (1983) A colour atlas of Bacillus species. Wolfe Medical Publications Ltd., London

Pomerantsev AP, Shishkova NA, Doronin IP, Sukovatova LV, Marinin LI (1993) Interaction of *Bacillus anthracis* with benzylpenicillin in vivo and in vitro. Antibiot Khimioter 38:30–33

Price LB, Hugh-Jones M, Jackson PJ, Keim P (1999) Genetic diversity in the protective antigen gene of *Bacillus anthracis*. J Bacteriol 181:2358–2362

Schupp J, Klevytska A, Zinser G, Price L, Keim P (2000) vrrB, a hypervariable open reading frame in *Bacillus anthracis*. J Bacteriol 182:3989–3997

Smith KL et al. (1999) Meso-scale ecology of anthrax in southern Africa: a pilot study of diversity and clustering. J Appl Microbiol 87:204–207

Sterne M (1937a) The effects of different carbon dioxide concentrations on the growth of virulent anthrax strains. Onderstepoort Journal of Veterinary Science and Animal Industry 9:49–67

Sterne M (1937b) Variation in *Bacillus anthracis*. Onderstepoort Journal of Veterinary Science and Animal Industry 8:271–349

Sterne M (1938) Variation in the colony form of the anthrax bacillus. Onderstepoort Journal of Veterinary Science and Animal Industry 10:245–250

Thorne C (1993) *Bacillus anthracis*. In: Sonenshein A (ed) *Bacillus subtilis* and Other Gram-Positive Bacteria. ASM Press, Washington, DC

Turnbull P (1998) Guidelines for the surveillance and control of anthrax in humans and animals, 3rd edn. World Health Organization, Geneva

Turner AJ, Galvin JW, Rubira RJ, Condron RJ, Bradley T (1999a) Experiences with vaccination and epidemiological investigations on an anthrax outbreak in Australia in 1997. J Appl Microbiol 87:294–297

Turner AJ, Galvin JW, Rubira RJ, Miller GT (1999b) Anthrax explodes in an Australian summer. J Appl Microbiol 87:196–199

CHAPTER 3

Anthrax Vaccines

A. M. FRIEDLANDER, S. L. WELKOS, B. E. IVINS

Abstract. The only impetus for the development of new anthrax vaccines is to protect humans against the intentional use of *Bacillus anthracis* as a bioterrorist or warfare agent. Live attenuated vaccines against anthrax in domesticated animals were among the very first vaccines developed. This was followed by the development of nonliving component vaccines leading to the eventual licensure of protein-based vaccines for human use in the 1970s. This chapter will review the recent advances in developing protein, live attenuated, and genetic vaccines against anthrax.

A. M. FRIEDLANDER, S. L. WELKOS, B. E. IVINS
U. S. Army Medical Research Institute of Infectious Diseases, 1425 Porter Street, Frederick, MD 21702, USA, Email: friedlander@amedd.army.mil.

1 Introduction

Anthrax has been associated with the very origins of microbiology and immunology in the latter part of the nineteenth century. Likewise, anthrax, an economically important disease of domesticated livestock at that time, was one of the first bacterial diseases against which an effective live vaccine was developed (Plotkin and Plotkin 1999). Live attenuated anthrax vaccines to protect animals have been in wide use since then. Similar live vaccines for human use were first developed in the former Soviet Union in the 1940s to protect against both naturally occurring disease and the threat of the use of *Bacillus anthracis* as a biological weapon (Shlyakhov and Rubinstein 1994). Non-living component or chemical vaccines for human use were developed in the 1950s in both the United States and the United Kingdom. Although the incidence of naturally occurring human anthrax is very low, there is clearly a resurgence of interest in developing new vaccines to protect people against anthrax arising from the use of *B. anthracis* as a bioterrorist or warfare agent. Recapitulating the earliest work on developing vaccines against anthrax and other infectious diseases, efforts are ongoing to develop both defined component as well as live attenuated vaccines. Although the main emphasis has been on protein vaccines, prepared with new adjuvants and delivery systems, there has also been recent interest in re-examining attenuated live vaccines and in applying the newer approaches of genetic vaccination to anthrax.

Our knowledge of the basis of immunity to human infection with *B. anthracis* is limited. Immunity after human cutaneous anthrax likely occurs, because reinfections are reported very rarely and tend to be much less severe (Hodgson 1941). Data in animals also suggest that animals surviving anthrax infection are more resistant to subsequent challenge (Wilson and Miles 1955). Immunity to infection can be induced by vaccination, and there is a large body of evidence showing that protection can be transferred with serum from animals vaccinated with spores (Gladstone 1946), culture filtrates (Belton and Strange 1954), or protective antigen (PA) alone (Little et al. 1997), suggesting that antibodies are the main mechanism of vaccine-induced immunity. Although the exact mechanisms of antibody-mediated protection against anthrax are not completely understood, recent progress in elucidating the pathogenesis of anthrax and the molecular basis of bacterial virulence have yielded advances with applications toward improved anthrax vaccine prophylaxis.

This chapter will briefly review the early work on vaccines and then will focus on the more recent efforts on developing new vaccines. More complete discussions of the early vaccines are available in several previous reviews (LINCOLN and FISH 1970; HAMBLETON et al. 1984; TURNBULL 1991).

2
Live Attenuated Vaccines

2.1
Early Live *Bacillus anthracis* Vaccines

The discovery by PASTEUR and GREENFIELD (TIGERTT 1980) of an in vitro procedure for reducing the virulence of *B. anthracis* by extended culture at elevated temperature was essential to the development of the first effective anthrax vaccine. PASTEUR's demonstration of protective vaccination of livestock against anthrax in 1881 (PASTEUR 1881) has been credited as one of the first documented uses of a bacterial vaccine and reinforced the concept of attenuation of virulent organisms as a general means of vaccination (PLOTKIN and PLOTKIN 1999). Vaccination with the Pasteur duplex vaccine required that two inoculations be given, using cultures of vegetative organisms grown at elevated temperature to obtain different levels of residual virulence. Although it was known that this process likely resulted in a mixed population of encapsulated fully virulent organisms together with attenuated variants (PRIESZ 1911), the probable mechanism of attenuation was not elucidated until the 1980s, when MIKESELL et al. (1983) showed that growing fully virulent strains at 42 °C cured the bacilli of the pX01 plasmid, which encodes the three proteins that compose the two anthrax toxins, lethal toxin and edema toxin. One of the proteins, protective antigen (PA), is an essential part of all effective live and nonliving component vaccines. Thus the Pasteur vaccines likely consisted of a mixture of varying amounts of nontoxinogenic encapsulated and toxinogenic encapsulated fully virulent strains. Although the Pasteur vaccine was effective and in widespread use in cattle and sheep for more than 50 years, variations in attenuation, instability, and inconvenient method of preparation led to its replacement with more stable attenuated spore vaccines.

The isolation by Sterne of an attenuated nonencapsulated toxinogenic (pX01+, pX02−) variant of *B. anthracis*, and its subsequent development as a live attenuated spore vaccine has had a great impact on controlling the disease in livestock (STERNE 1937; STERNE et al. 1942). Although this vaccine appears to be very effective and safe for use in domestic animals, it clearly has a low but significant level of virulence in laboratory animals, including guinea pigs and mice (TURNBULL et al 1986; WELKOS and FRIEDLANDER 1988; IVINS et al. 1990a) and in some domesticated animals (TURNBULL 1991). Concern for the potential safety and reactogenicity of the live vaccine has been a factor in impeding the use in Western countries of such live vaccines in humans. However, a Sterne-like strain, STI-1, was licensed for human use in 1953 in the former Soviet Union (SHLYAKHOV and RUBINSTEIN 1994). It is administered subcutaneously or by scarification of the skin, and epidemiological studies reported its efficacy against cutaneous disease (SHUYLAK 1970; SHLYAKHOV and RUBINSTEIN 1994). Aerosol vaccination in humans has also been reported to generate an immune response and be reasonably well tolerated (GEFEN et al. 1970; SHLYAKHOV and RUBINSTEIN 1994).

Despite their potential reactogenicity compared with nonliving component vaccines, live vaccines have often demonstrated superior protection in experimental animal models in regard to time to onset of immunity, the number of doses required to achieve effective immunity, the duration of protection, and the breadth of coverage. These attributes have been the impetus behind the continued research on developing new-generation live vaccines that are safe, easy to administer, and effective. For instance, studies in guinea pigs compared the spore vaccine to the US-licensed vaccine, Anthrax Vaccine Adsorbed (AVA), and the UK vaccine. They showed that the spore vaccine is more protective than the cell-free vaccine (IVINS et al. 1986; LITTLE and KNUDSON 1986; TURNBULL et al. 1986; IVINS and WELKOS 1988; BROSTER and HIBBS 1990). This occurs despite the often lower titer of anti-PA antibodies in live- compared with AVA-vaccinated animals. Other studies showed that vaccination with PA followed by a booster with the live Sterne vaccine confers significantly greater protection than does a booster with PA (KLEIN et al. 1962).

The evidence for the superiority of live attenuated over component vaccines must be qualified, as some of the differences reported may depend on the experimental design and the adjuvant used. In one study, a single large dose of PA was significantly more protective earlier than a live vaccine (KLEIN et al. 1962). It should also be noted that the observations of the superiority of live vaccines have been made mainly in guinea pigs with aluminum adjuvants. When guinea pigs were vaccinated with PA prepared with other adjuvants, the animals were as completely protected as they were by the live spore vaccine (Ivins et al. 1992). Thus it is possible that an equivalent degree of immunity may be attained with better adjuvants and delivery systems using larger amounts of more immunologically potent native antigens. The protection afforded cattle vaccinated with two doses of PA and aluminum potassium sulfate (alum) was not significantly different from that in animals given a single dose of a live spore vaccine (Jackson et al. 1957). It has also been reported that rabbits (Auerbach and Wright 1955; Fellows et al. 2001) and nonhuman primates (Fellows et al. 2001) given nonliving component vaccines prepared with aluminum adjuvants develop a much higher degree of protection than do guinea pigs against a more geographically diverse group of strains. Nevertheless, it remains possible that the improved immunity reported with live vaccines may be real and, as previously suggested (Ivins and Welkos 1988), due to factors such as prolonged exposure to protective immunogens presented in a more native conformation. In addition, live vaccines may contain additional protective immunogens present in the spore or bacillus that are lacking in the component vaccines and thus may more closely reproduce the immunity generated by a natural infection.

Several approaches have been used in efforts to create new live vaccines. In general, these strains have been developed to be further attenuated than the toxinogenic [pX01+], nonencapsulated [pX02–], Sterne-type vaccines, which have been considered too reactogenic for human use. These approaches include generation of attenuating mutations in Sterne strains, use of recombinant *B. anthracis* strains, use of organisms other than *B. anthracis* as carriers of protective antigen, and genetic vaccination strategies.

2.2 *Bacillus anthracis* Aro-Mutants

Aromatic compound-dependent mutants of a toxinogenic, nonencapsulated strain of *B. anthracis* (Aro-) were isolated by mutagenesis with the tetracycline resistance transposon *Tn*916. They were greatly attenuated for mice and guinea pigs and protected these difficult-to-protect species against the virulent Ames strain with up to 80% of the former and 100% of the latter surviving challenge (Ivins and Welkos 1988; Ivins et al. 1990a). However, their further consideration as live vaccine candidates would require the elimination of their self-transmitting tetracycline resistance factor and their ability to revert to the Aro^+ Tc^s phenotype. Such strains with defined mutations in the relevant genes in the aromatic amino acid pathway deserve further evaluation as vaccines.

2.3
Toxin-Deficient Mutants of *Bacillus anthracis*

Mock and coworkers constructed and characterized derivatives of the Sterne strain that were deficient in each of the three toxin proteins (Pezard et al. 1991, 1993, 1995). The toxin genes for PA (*pag*), edema factor (EF) (*cya*), and lethal factor (LF) (*lef*) were inactivated by a large internal deletion in the coding region and insertion of an antibiotic-resistance cassette (Erm^r or Kan^r). These constructs were prepared in *Escherichia coli* and transferred to the *B. anthracis* recipient by use of a conjugal transfer system and mobilizable shuttle plasmid. Strains were isolated that had lost the introduced plasmid vector and, by homologous recombination, had replaced the wild-type toxin gene on pX01 with the corresponding deleted copy with the inserted antibiotic-resistance cassette. These mutant strains have provided useful insights into the roles of each of the anthrax toxins in disease pathogenesis and in immune protection. The advantage of this system was the creation of mutants that retained the native copy number of the altered gene in its pX01 location and still subject to its usual genetic environment and regulatory state. A drawback of the use of these constructs as vaccines is the retention of the antibiotic-resistance genes.

In the studies of Cataldi, Pezard, and coworkers with these mutant strains (Cataldi et al. 1990; Pezard et al. 1991), they found that the mutant that produced PA and LF but was EF negative, although less virulent than the parental strain, still caused a lethal infection. This supports the idea that lethal toxin is a key virulence factor required for lethality. Skin edema was produced with the LF^- mutant that secreted only PA and EF, although this strain was less virulent than that producing only lethal toxin [PA+, LF+, EF–]. However, the parental Sterne strain producing all three components was more lethal and caused more edema than the mutants producing the single toxins. This provides supporting evidence that the toxins are synergistic in their effects in vivo. Although this general statement is true, it may reflect the fact that the strain producing both toxins, being more virulent, may be more metabolically active, producing more edema toxin and thus generating more edema, rather than that the individual protein toxins by themselves are synergistic in producing edema. This finding, nevertheless, supports older studies performed with partially purified toxin components (Smith and Stoner 1967). Elucidation of the mechanism of the postulated synergism between the toxins will require further studies with highly pure individual proteins. Finally, all strains of *B. anthracis*, including ones cured of both pX01 and pX02, survive longer than *B. subtilis* in the mouse, thus implicating a role for chromosomally encoded genes in the pathogenesis of infection. This persistence may be due in part to the resistance of *B. anthracis* but not *B. subtilis* to lysis by lysozyme present in mammalian tissue (Gordon et al. 1973).

Pezard et al. extended the genetic methodology developed originally to isolate mutant strains deficient in one toxin component (Cataldi et al. 1990; Pezard et al. 1991) to construct double mutants that produce only the single toxin components PA, EF, or LF (Pezard et al. 1993). Subcutaneous infection of mice with these strains (10^9 cfu) proved conclusively that individually none of the three proteins secreted by the organisms in vivo is toxic for animals, a finding consistent with previous results obtained after injection of the proteins into animals (Cataldi et al. 1990). One caveat to these findings is the use of the attenuated Sterne strain as the virulent challenge strain. This nonencapsulated strain has an LD_{50} for mice (10^6 spores) that is 10^5- to 10^6-fold higher than that of a fully virulent, pX01$^+$ pX02$^+$ strain of *B. anthracis*, requiring the injection of $\geq 10^9$ cfu of the test strain to show an attenuating effect.

The antibody responses to infection and the level of protection from lethal anthrax challenge induced by all six mutant strains (deficient in 1 or 2 of the toxin component proteins) of *B. anthracis* were compared (Pezard et al. 1995). High anti-PA titers were obtained after inoculation with the strain producing only PA. However, titers to LF and EF were low in mice inoculated with LF- or EF-producing mutants that were PA-negative. These titers were significantly higher in animals inoculated with the bacteria also producing PA, suggesting an adjuvant role for PA in stimulation of anti-LF/-EF antibodies. Comparing the levels of protection against a lethal Sterne challenge in mice vaccinated with the different toxin mutants confirmed the role of PA as the major protective antigen but provided conflicting evidence for the role of LF and EF in immunoprotection. The results are somewhat surprising in that protection with a strain producing only LF was equivalent to that observed with a strain producing only PA. This contrasts with the small amount of published data with the isolated proteins that showed that PA alone is protective whereas LF alone confers minimal or no protection against challenge with fully virulent toxinogenic encapsulated organisms (Little and Knudson 1986; Ivins and Welkos 1988; see below). There was also a suggestion in some but not all experimental groups that strains containing PA plus LF or PA plus EF were more protective than a strain producing PA alone. This is consistent with some older studies but not the more recent data obtained by using purified proteins and confirms that this remains an unresolved issue requiring further study (see below). These results may reflect the fact that the challenge organism used in these live vaccine studies was the less virulent unencapsulated Sterne strain, which is easier to protect against, or perhaps that the toxin proteins produced by the live strain in vivo were more protective than those purified from in vitro-grown organisms. In addition, the toxin proteins produced in vivo from live strains may form complexes that are more protective than vaccines composed of the separate uncomplexed protein components adsorbed to aluminum hydroxide. Finally, because PA-negative mutants still provided some protection, whereas the pX01-cured derivative of Sterne was completely nonprotective and probably failed to replicate in vivo, it is possible that the protection afforded by the PA-deficient strains may have been due to an immune response to pX01-encoded nontoxin antigens of *B. anthracis* (Hibbs 1990). Similar experiments with a pX01-containing strain with deletions in *pag, lef, and cya* would be of interest, as would testing of these various strains against challenge with a fully virulent strain.

Brossier et al. (Brossier et al. 1999a, 2000) developed a genetic approach to isolating toxin-deficient attenuated mutants of *B. anthracis* that yielded strains with features that made them better suited as candidate live vaccines. In contrast to the initial deletion-insertion strategy to construct toxin-deficient strains, the more recent approach allowed the introduction of a defined point mutation or partial deletion into pX01 without additional heterologous DNA, i.e., vector sequences and/or antibiotic-resistance cassettes. This strategy was used to create strains with mutations to disrupt the functional domains of PA involving binding of PA to the host cell receptor, LF/EF binding, and their translocation to the cytosol. Also, mutations were introduced to knock out the metalloprotease activity of LF and adenylate cyclase activity of EF. These mutants were all significantly attenuated in the mouse/Sterne challenge model, thus verifying that the functional domains on PA and the metalloprotease activity of LF and adenylate cyclase activity of EF, as defined and studied in vitro, were required for lethality and edema formation, respectively. However, strains producing lethal toxin and expressing an inactive EF, or producing edema toxin and expressing an inactive LF, were significantly less virulent and less effective at producing lethality and edema, respectively, than were the unmutated parental strains. These findings are consistent with the previous suggestion that the toxins act synergistically to produce lethality and edema in vivo (PEZARD et al. 1995) but might also be explained by the fact that the strain producing both toxins, being more virulent, is more metabolically active, producing more toxin, in vivo, than the mutants.

Immunogenicity studies confirmed, as suggested previously (PEZARD et al. 1991), that the extent of the antibody response to LF induced by vaccination with the mutants was dependent on the presence of PA. It was further found that the binding of LF to PA was necessary and sufficient for a good antibody response to LF. Neither LF enzymatic activity nor binding of the lethal toxin complex (PA + LF) to the host cell receptor was needed to induce high-titer anti-LF antibody. These results suggesting that PA and LF form a complex without interacting with cell receptors for PA are consistent with previous observations showing that complexes of PA and LF exist in serum in vivo (EZZELL and ABSHIRE 1992).

The strain synthesizing wild-type PA and inactive LF and EF appeared to be an especially attractive live vaccine candidate because it is isogenic to the effective Sterne animal vaccine while being fully attenuated, yet retains all the immunogens possessed by Sterne (BROSSIER et al. 2000). Its efficacy was shown by the protection of all mice vaccinated with one dose of the mutant against challenge with 40 LD_{50} of a virulent encapsulated strain of *B. anthracis*. It would be interesting to carefully compare its efficacy with that of the parental Sterne strain and against inhalational anthrax in animal models with a pathology and course of disease more closely resembling that of humans (IVINS et al. 1996; PITT et al. 1996b, 1999). This may help answer the question of whether an immune response directed at the active sites of LF and EF contributes at all to protection.

2.4 *Bacillus anthracis* Recombinant Vaccines

Live recombinant *B. anthracis*-based vaccines have been constructed and characterized. Barnard and Friedlander (BARNARD and FRIEDLANDER 1999) transformed two nonencapsulated, nontoxinogenic strains of *B. anthracis*, ΔANR and ΔSterne, with various shuttle vectors expressing different levels of PA. The shuttle vectors consisted of either the gram-positive vector pUB110 or pC194 ligated to an *E. coli* vector containing the PA gene from *B. anthracis* strain Sterne. These constructs provided tools for assessing the effects of chromosomal background and of the amount of PA produced on vaccine efficacy against the fully virulent Ames strain. No significant strain-related effects were found on PA production in vitro, plasmid stability in vivo, survival of the vaccination strain in the host (guinea pig), or protective efficacy. The level of protection of the recombinant strains correlated with the anti-PA antibody titers induced in vivo, demonstrating for the first time a direct correlation of antibody with immunity. Protection also correlated with the level of PA the strains produced in vitro. In contrast to the lethality in guinea pigs and mice given doses of $\geq 10^7$ spores of Sterne and STI-1 (TURNBULL et al 1986; WELKOS and FRIEDLANDER 1988; IVINS et al. 1990), a single dose of 10^9 spores of either the ΔANR (pPA102) or ΔSterne (pPA102) live vaccine strains was nonlethal in the guinea pig model and as effective in these animals as one dose of the licensed human anthrax vaccine. These results suggested that increasing the level of PA production would enhance the efficacy of a live vaccine. This is consistent with the corollary hypothesis, namely, that decreasing the degradation of PA in a live vaccine might enhance its immunity. The latter possibility was first suggested by the earlier observations of FUBRA (1966), who showed that nonproteolytic mutants of the live Sterne vaccine strain, which might be expected to produce greater amounts of PA, were more protective than the parent strain.

Similar live vaccines were described subsequently by COHEN et al. (2000), who also constructed recombinant derivatives of a nonencapsulated, nontoxinogenic strain of *B. anthracis* that differed in their level of expression of PA cloned in shuttle vectors. The PA structural gene, *pag*, from Sterne was cloned into an *E. coli* vector, and variants having *pag* under the control of either the native *pag* promoter or the promoter of α-amylase gene of *B. amyloliquefaciens* (*Pa-amy*) were constructed. Shuttle vectors containing the two rPA-expressing constructs were used to transform strains of *B. subtilis* and of a pX01-cured *B. anthracis* deficient in extracellular proteases. Especially high levels of PA were obtained in those with the *Pa-amy* promoter. In the *B. anthracis* variant with this promoter, levels of secreted PA were tenfold higher than those expressed by *pag* with the native promoter. In contrast to the residual virulence of the licensed live vaccine (see above), doses of up to 10^9 spores of the PA-producing *B. anthracis* recombinant were nonlethal and could be used safely to vaccinate guinea pigs. A single dose of 5×10^7 spores of the latter strain induced high, persistent levels of neutralizing anti-PA antibodies and provided long-lasting protection of guinea pigs against a lethal parenteral challenge of *B. anthracis* strain Vollum. At high doses of the vaccine, there appeared to be a correlation between the level of expression of PA and the vaccine efficacy. However, a tenfold lower dose of spores failed to induce detectable titers of anti-PA antibodies yet protected against lethal challenge. Furthermore, a strain that lacks pX01 and does not produce PA provided some protection against virulent challenge. These results contrast with those of Pezard et al. (1995) cited above and Ivins et al. (1986). However, the findings are difficult to compare because different animal models, vaccination schedules, and challenge organisms were used in the various studies. Nevertheless, these results suggest a role for nontoxin antigens in eliciting protective immunity and suggest that there may be chromosomal genes contributing to immunity that differ between strains. To fully evaluate the efficacy of these new live recombinant candidate vaccines (Barnard and Friedlander 1999; Cohen et al. 2000), they should be tested against a lethal *B. anthracis* aerosol challenge in rabbits or nonhuman primates (Ivins et al. 1996; Pitt et al. 1996, 1999).

More recent work by Friedlander and coworkers (unpublished observations) showed significantly enhanced efficacy of the high PA-producing live recombinant strains by using an isogenic strain that also contains pX02 and produces capsule. The mechanism of the increased efficacy of this strain remains to be determined, but the results suggest that the capsule may increase the protection of live attenuated or protein vaccines containing PA.

2.5
Non-*Bacillus anthracis* Live Vaccine Carriers of Anthrax Toxin Antigens

The cloning and delivery of the PA vaccine antigen was also achieved with *B. subtilis* (Ivins and Welkos 1986; Welkos and Friedlander 1988; Welkos et al. 1990). The PA gene from *B. anthracis* was cloned in the gram-positive vector pUB110 (Ivins and Welkos 1986) and the latter transformed into the asporogenic *B. subtilis* strain IS53. Unlike recombinant *E. coli*, in which cloned proteins can often only be detected in culture lysates, PA is secreted by *B. subtilis* and can be isolated from the supernatant. The *B. subtilis* recombinants produced PA at levels equal to or greater than those of the *B. anthracis* strain Sterne. The pUB110-PA recombinant plasmid pPA101 was subsequently transferred to the sporogenic *B. subtilis* DB104 strain, and the clone PA7 was isolated. The *B.*

subtilis isolates were nonlethal at high doses in mice and guinea pigs, e.g., injection of $\leq 10^9$ cfu failed to kill guinea pigs although 10^7 cfu of Sterne spores produced >30% fatalities (WELKOS and FRIEDLANDER 1988; IVINS et al. 1990a). The PA-encoding *B. subtilis* strains strongly protected guinea pigs and mice against parenteral challenge with the fully virulent Ames strain, with 95%–100% of the former and 70% of the latter surviving (IVINS et al. 1990a, b; WELKOS et al. 1990).

Attenuated strains of *Salmonella typhimurium*, such as the *aroA* strain, have been used to deliver heterologous antigens and as live oral vaccines (CHATFIELD et al. 1994; SCHODEL and CURTISS 1995). Because of the ability of these organisms to invade the gut via the lymphoid tissues, such vaccines have the potential to induce mucosal as well as humoral and cell-mediated immune responses. COULSON et al. (1994) investigated the ability of live oral *Salmonella aroA* strains expressing PA to induce protective immunity against anthrax. The PA gene and upstream sequences were cloned into the gram-negative vector pBLSKIIl, and the recombinant strain given orally to mice partially protected against lethal challenge with *B. anthracis* strain Vollum 1B. Despite the absence of a serum anti-PA antibody response in the *S. typhimurium*-vaccinated mice, the protection afforded by the *aroA* recombinant (33%) was comparable to that achieved with PA combined with Ribi or incomplete Freund's adjuvants (25%–37%). These adjuvants protect mice and guinea pigs better than do aluminum-adjuvant containing PA vaccines (TURNBULL et al. 1986, 1990; IVINS et al. 1990b, 1992). Further investigations are warranted on the protective efficacy and nature of the immune response elicited by such heterologous oral live anthrax vaccines.

Other bacterial carriers were recently developed to express PA for use as live vaccines. These include *Lactobacillus casei*, which has been developed for use as an oral vaccine delivery system (ZEGERS et al. 1998). To date, the expression level of PA in this strain has been low and there are no data on its efficacy in animal models. A live attenuated vaccine strain of *Francisella tularensis* has also been engineered to express PA. Preliminary reports suggest that this strain is immunogenic in mice (Pavlov et al., unpublished data).

Viral vectors have also been used to clone and deliver *B. anthracis* immunogens. For example, recombinant PA-producing vaccinia (strain WR) elicited high anti-PA antibody titers in mice and provided significant protection of mice (60%) and guinea pigs (50%) against parenteral challenge with the fully virulent Ames strain (IACONO-CONNORS et al. 1991).

3 Genetic Vaccination

Over the past decade, vaccination with DNA has been applied to many different diseases. Recent studies have shown that intramuscular vaccination with DNA encoding the PA of anthrax toxin induced toxin-neutralizing antibodies and protected mice against death from low doses of lethal toxin (Gu et al. 1999). No studies were done to test the vaccine against infection. Other workers reported that DNA encoding PA can effectively prime mice to a booster with the PA protein (Williamson et al. 1999). Studies performed in guinea pigs with a similar DNA plasmid encoding PA showed that four doses of DNA given by gene gun induced low levels of antibody and failed to protect the animals against an intramuscular challenge with 100 LD_{50} of a virulent *B. anthracis* strain. More recent experiments showed that a vaccination with a single priming dose of DNA followed by two booster doses with PA given with the Ribi adjuvant system protected five of six animals against a similar challenge with virulent organisms (C. Schmaljohn, personal communication). This degree of protection was similar to that observed in the group of animals vaccinated with the PA given with adjuvant alone (6 of 6 animals survived), although the antibody titers were slightly lower. Other groups found that plasmids containing DNA encoding for LF, as well as those encoding for PA, protect mice against lethal toxin challenge (D. Galloway, personal communication). This is consistent with previous observations that antibodies to LF can neutralize toxin in vitro and protect animals from death induced by the lethal toxin (Little et al. 1990). Furthermore, mice were protected against challenge with the attenuated *B. anthracis* strain Sterne with DNA encoding for PA or PA and LF as a priming dose followed by protein boosters (L. Baillie and D. Galloway, personal communication).

Alternative strategies of genetic vaccination have included the use of nonreplicating RNA viruses encoding for PA. A Venezuelan equine encephalitis (VEE) virus replicon-based vaccine delivery system was developed to facilitate the expression of heterologous proteins and stimulate an immune response in vivo (Pushko et al. 1997). This system is composed of a self-replicating RNA expression vector (replicon) containing all of the VEE virus nonstructural genes and the PA gene in place of the VEE structural genes. Cotransfection of cells in vitro with a replicon and two helper RNA molecules, which encode the structural proteins, results in the production of propagation-deficient VEE replicon particles (VRPs). Cells infected with VRPs encoding PA expressed high levels of the protein in vitro. Mice inoculated subcutaneously with three doses of VRPs encoding PA were completely protected against subcutaneous challenge with the attenuated *B. anthracis* strain Sterne (J. L. Lee, personal communication). Protection correlated directly with serum ELISA titers to PA. The VEE replicons have been used to express other antigens as well as PA and appear to be a potentially useful multivalent vaccine delivery and expression vehicle. Further studies are being pursued to determine the ability of the VRPs (encoding PA and possibly other *B. anthracis* immunogens) to protect animals against challenge with fully virulent strains and by the aerosol route as well.

Genetic vaccination as well as the use of different adjuvants with protein antigens (see below) offer the potential of stimulating both humoral and cellular immunity, although it remains to be seen whether the latter is important in resistance to anthrax.

4
Protein Component Vaccines

The early development of vaccines against anthrax went through a similar evolution, as did vaccines to protect against other infectious diseases. The use of nonliving component vaccines followed the original studies showing protection with live attenuated strains of *B. anthracis*. Bail in 1904 (1904) and, subsequently, Salsbery in 1926 (1926) were the first to report protection against anthrax, not with live strains of *B. anthracis* but with edematous fluid from infected animals. This material undoubtedly contained the then-unknown PA as well as EF and LF. In the 1940s Cromartie et al. (1947) and Watson et al. (1947) extended these studies to show protection in several species. Gladstone (1946), following on studies of others, demonstrated the presence of a "protective antigen" produced in cultures of *B. anthracis* that was capable of immunizing a number of animal species against lethal *B. anthracis* challenge. It was the work of Wright, Puziss, and colleagues in the United States (Wright et al. 1954; Auerbach and Wright 1955; Puziss and Wright 1962; Puziss et al. 1963) and Belton, Strange, and colleagues in England (Belton and Strange 1954; Lincoln and Fish 1970) during the 1950s and 1960s that led to the development of the first US and UK human anthrax vaccines, respectively.

4.1 Human Vaccines

The licensed US human anthrax vaccine (Anthrax Vaccine Adsorbed, or AVA) has been approved by the United States Food and Drug Administration since 1970. It consists of aluminum hydroxide-adsorbed supernatant material, most importantly PA, from synthetic medium fermentor cultures of a nonencapsulated, toxinogenic strain of *B. anthracis*, V770-NP1-R. The vaccine contains formaldehyde as a stabilizing agent and benzethonium chloride as a preservative (Puziss and Wright 1962). The vaccine is administered subcutaneously in 0.5-ml doses at 0, 2, and 4 weeks and then at 6, 12, and 18 months, with yearly boosters thereafter (Brachman and Friedlander 1999). A recent study found that a schedule of doses at 0 and 4 weeks, eliminating the 2-week dose, resulted in an equivalent anti-PA antibody response at 6–24 weeks compared with the 0-, 2-, and 4-week schedule, suggesting it may be possible to eliminate one of the doses (P.R. Pittman, personal communication). The vaccine is recommended for individuals at occupational risk of anthrax, specifically, those who work with animals and animal products such as hides, wool, or bones and those who work with *B. anthracis* in the laboratory. In 1998, members of the US Armed Forces began to receive the vaccine in response to concerns that *B. anthracis* spores might be used as a biological weapon (Friedlander et al. 1999). There are no human efficacy data for the current anthrax vaccine. However, there are clinical data from the use of a less potent precursor of the licensed AVA that employed alum-precipitated supernatant material from cultures of the *B. anthracis* Vollum R1-NP strain (Brachman et al. 1962). A significant degree of protection (93%) was demonstrated in a placebo-controlled study carried out in goat hair mill workers in the Northeastern United States during 1955–58. There was 1 case of cutaneous anthrax in the vaccinated group compared with 13 cutaneous and 2 inhalational cases of anthrax in the unvaccinated placebo group. There were three additional cases of inhalational anthrax in unvaccinated workers who did not take part in the study and none in the vaccinated group (Brachman et al. 1962). The data on the safety and efficacy of the AVA were recently reviewed (Brachman and Friedlander 1999; Friedlander et al. 1999).

AVA has been tested for efficacy in several laboratory animal models, and it is important to bear in mind that efficacy varies significantly with the test animal. This vaccine is highly efficacious against virulent *B.*

anthracis spore challenge in both rabbits and nonhuman primates exposed to aerosols of the agent (IVINS et al. 1996, 1998; PITT et al. 1996, 1999 FELLOWS et al. 2001); nonhuman primates are believed to be the best model of human disease and to best reflect the immune response of humans. In guinea pigs, AVA provides varying degrees of protection against a parenteral challenge and it is very difficult to provide good protection against an aerosol challenge (IVINS et al. 1992, 1994, 1995; FELLOWS et al. 2001). It is noteworthy that the efficacy of PA vaccines can be increased significantly in guinea pigs by using adjuvants other than aluminum (see below). This suggests that the difficulty in protecting the guinea pig is due to its inability to respond to aluminum adjuvants rather than that the PA does not protect. Furthermore, the protection induced by AVA varies depending on the strain of *B. anthracis* used for challenge (FELLOWS et al. 2001; IVINS et al. 1994). However, strains of *B. anthracis* that are highly virulent ("vaccine resistant") in AVA-vaccinated guinea pigs do not have the same ability to overcome vaccination in other species. Thus rabbits and nonhuman primates challenged with isolates from various geographic locations, including those that overcome AVA vaccination in guinea pigs, were all protected by vaccination with AVA (FELLOWS et al. 2001). Indeed, no *B. anthracis* strain has been identified that is "vaccine-resistant" in rabbits or monkeys.

Hamsters are not protected at all (FELLOWS et al. 2000), whereas in mice the efficacy of AVA is poor at best (WELKOS et al. 1990; IVINS et al. 1992). Strains of *B. anthracis* that produce only capsule and are avirulent in other animals (IVINS et al. 1986) are virulent in mice (WELKOS et al. 1993), so that the virulence factors also vary between species.

The human anthrax vaccine in the United Kingdom was originally developed in the 1950s and licensed in 1979 (TURNBULL 2000). This vaccine differs somewhat from the US vaccine. Static cultures of the Sterne 34F2 strain of *B. anthracis* are grown in protein hydrolysate medium, and then alum is used to precipitate supernatant material. With respect to protective efficacy in experimental animals, it behaves quite similarly to AVA (TURNBULL et al. 1986, 1988). In contrast to AVA, the UK vaccine induces high levels of anti-LF antibodies and lower levels of antibodies to EF in humans (TURNBULL et al. 1986, 1988). Low levels of antibody to LF have been reported in guinea pigs after vaccination with AVA (TURNBULL et al. 1986; IVINS and WELKOS 1988).

4.2 New Protein Vaccines

PA is the singularly most important antigen required for specific immunity to anthrax. In 1986 it was demonstrated definitively for the first time with PA cloned into *B. subtilis* that no other antigen from *B. anthracis* is needed for protective immunity (Ivins and Welkos 1986). However, the presence of other antigens, particularly EF or LF, may augment protection, as evidenced by data from experiments with the guinea pig animal model (Stanley and Smith 1963; Berendt et al. 1985; Ivins and Welkos 1988), as discussed below. PA is a protein with a molecular weight of 83,000 (Leppla 1996; Little and Ivins 1999), but the entire molecule is not necessary for a vaccine to engender protection. Indeed, proteolysis by trypsin cleaves the PA molecule into polypeptides of 63,000 and 20,000 Da; the former but not the latter is protectively immunogenic in a guinea pig challenge model (Ivins and Welkos 1988). In the host, a trypsin-like protease, likely furin on the host cell surface and/or a serum protease, cleaves PA to reveal the site on the 63,000-Da fragment responsible for binding EF or LF, generating edema toxin or lethal toxin, respectively. In addition to the EF/LF binding site, PA also possesses a site in domain 4 in the C terminus of the protein (Petosa et al. 1997) responsible for binding of the molecule to the host cell receptor (Little et al. 1996; Singh et al. 1991; Brossier et al. 1999b; Varughese et al. 1999). These two binding sites may well contain those antigenic epitopes most critical to inducing a protective immune response to anthrax. In live attenuated strains, the cell receptor-binding domain of PA, in contrast to the EF/LF binding site, is more important in generating an antibody response to PA (Brossier et al. 2000). A PA mutant that could not be cleaved by the cell protease in vitro (and presumably in vivo) so that the EF/LF binding site was not exposed, was protective when used as a vaccine (Singh et al. 1998). However, no quantitative comparison with intact PA was made. It has been established that vaccination with PA induces antibodies to both the cell receptor and the EF/LF binding domains that neutralize the cytotoxicity of lethal toxin in vitro (Little et al. 1997). The relative importance in vaccine efficacy of these two functional domains on PA requires a more definitive study. Other domains on PA, including those responsible for oligomerization and translocation to the cytosol (Novak et al. 1992; Singh et al. 1999; Sellman et al. 2000), might also prove to contain protective epitopes if they are readily exposed to antibody in vivo.

Considerable research effort has been devoted during the past two decades to developing a new human anthrax vaccine (IVINS and WELKOS 1988; TURNBULL 1991). The only reason to develop a new vaccine is to protect against disease arising as a result of the intentional release of *B. anthracis* spores by a bioterrorist or in warfare, because the incidence of human disease, particularly inhalational anthrax, is extraordinarily low. A major objective in developing a new vaccine would be to induce protective immunity using fewer doses than required with the current licensed vaccine.

The research effort to develop newer anthrax protein vaccines began in several laboratories throughout the world shortly after 1980. The finding by MIKESELL and coworkers in 1983 that PA is encoded on a large plasmid (pXO1) (MIKESELL et al. 1983) led eventually to the PA gene being cloned into *E. coli* (VODKIN and LEPPLA 1983), subcloned into *B. subtilis* (IVINS and WELKOS 1986), and electroporated back into a plasmid-free *B. anthracis* strain, ΔSterne-1. The resulting strain, *B. anthracis* ΔSterne-1(pPA102), produced PA at high levels, but no LF, EF, or capsule (FARCHAUS et al. 1998). This provided a source of PA free of the other toxin components that was used in animal studies to confirm that PA alone was protective (IVINS et al. 1998). An asporogenic mutant of this strain was isolated and is currently used to produce the recombinant PA (rPA) for incorporation into candidate human anthrax vaccines in the United States (WORSHAM and SOWERS 1999). MILLER et al. (1998) cloned the PA gene into *B. subtilis* WB600 and showed the purified PA to be protective in guinea pigs. IACONO-CONNORS et al. (1991) cloned rPA into baculovirus and demonstrated that the purified protein was as efficacious as *B. anthracis* PA in the guinea pig model. Recombinant PA was also produced and purified from *E. coli* (COULSON et al. 1994; BENSON et al. 1998; GUPTA et al. 1999) and from *B. brevis* (OH et al. 1998). PA from an *E. coli* construct was equivalent to PA produced by *B. anthracis* in protecting rabbits from aerosol challenge (Ivins et al., unpublished observations).

For many years, investigators have sought to determine whether EF or LF confers any additional protection when added to a PA vaccine. Early studies by STANLEY and SMITH (1963) suggested that EF may enhance the immunity produced by PA, whereas studies by MAHLANDT et al. (1966) were quite complex and gave conflicting results. Both studies used impure preparations, and the results were difficult to interpret. Later investigators found either no effect of EF or LF (LITTLE and KNUDSON 1986) or only an effect, which did not reach statistical significance, suggesting that both

EF and LF increase the efficacy of PA alone (BERENDT et al. 1985; IVINS and WELKOS 1988). These limited studies left the question unresolved, and a definitive answer will require additional research using larger challenge doses in different animal models.

There has been little work on antigens other than the toxin components, although as noted above the putative increased protection of live vaccines suggests that they may exist. In a single study, vaccination with preparations containing the S-layer protein EA1 and cell wall polysaccharides did not protect animals against challenge with virulent strains (EZZELL and ABSHIRE 1988). The possible effect of the capsule on contributing to protective immunity was described above in preliminary experiments showing that a live vaccine producing capsule was more protective than an isogenic strain making only PA (Friedlander, unpublished observations). Older work based on passive protection studies with ill-defined serum suggested that antibodies to the capsule can protect mice but not rabbits (WILSON and MILES 1955).

4.3 New Vaccine Adjuvants

Work in several laboratories over the last two decades has demonstrated the importance of the adjuvant or carrier selected for a new candidate anthrax vaccine. In numerous experiments IVINS and coworkers combined PA with one of several adjuvants and then tested the vaccine preparations for efficacy in mice, guinea pigs, rabbits, or rhesus monkeys (IVINS et al. 1990, 1992, 1995, 1998; PITT et al. 1996a). The adjuvant in AVA, aluminum hydroxide (Alhydrogel), is a potent stimulator of the Th2 humoral immune response, but not a Th1 cellular immune response (GUPTA and SIBER 1995). It was effective when combined with PA in protecting rabbits and monkeys from virulent aerosol spore challenge. However, Alhydrogel + PA, like AVA, provides insignificant protection to mice from a parenteral challenge and failed to protect hamsters (FELLOWS et al. 2000). Guinea pigs were afforded variable protection against either parenteral or aerosol spore challenge by vaccination with PA adsorbed to Alhydrogel (IVINS et al. 1992, 1994, 1995; FELLOWS et al. 2001). It is noteworthy that, although there are vast differences in protection among the different species, a strong specific antibody response to PA was engendered in all the species vaccinated with Alhydrogel + PA. The differences in protection seen suggest two possible explanations: (1) the specific mechanisms of immunity to anthrax may vary among species; or (2) the ability of Alhydrogel + PA to stimulate a highly protective immune response may be greater in some species than in others. Other workers primarily use guinea pigs in their anthrax vaccine efficacy studies, and their results with both the US and UK vaccines indicate that guinea pigs are afforded variable levels of protection by vaccination with either product (Turnbull et al. 1986, 1988, 1990).

In AVA, formalin is added as a stabilizer (Puziss and Wright 1962). Recent studies in guinea pigs suggest that adding formalin to Alhydrogel + PA may actually enhance the potency of the vaccine (Ivins, unpublished observations). The specific mechanism is as yet undetermined, but it may be that formalin acts on the PA to either expose or stabilize critical protective epitopes. It is also possible that formalin itself has adjuvant properties, by increasing the local inflammatory response to PA.

Aluminum salts such as aluminum hydroxide, aluminum potassium sulfate (alum), and aluminum phosphate are currently the only adjuvants approved for use in human vaccines. Numerous experimental adjuvants and carriers in addition to aluminum hydroxide were recently tested in laboratory animals with PA or with either the US or UK human anthrax vaccine (Ivins et al. 1988, 1992, 1995, 1998; Turnbull et al. 1990; McBride et al. 1998; Fellows et al. 2000). These include: (1) the lipid amine CP-20,961 (Ivins et al. 1992); (2) saponin QS-21 (Ivins et al. 1995, 1998); (3) MF-59 emulsion (Ivins et al. 1995); (4) SAF-M emulsion containing pluronic block copolymer L121 (Ivins et al. 1995); (5) muramyl tripeptide (MTP) (Ivins et al. 1995, 1998); (6) threonyl muramyl dipeptide (T-MDP) (Ivins et al. 1992, 1995); (7) monophosphoryl lipid A (MPL) (Ivins et al. 1992, 1995, 1998); (8) the combination of MPL with trehalose dimycolate (TDM) and mycobacterial cell wall skeleton (CWS) (Ivins et al. 1992; Turnbull 1991; McBride et al. 1998); (9) MPL + CWS (Ivins et al. 1992); (10) heat-killed *Corynebacterium ovis* (Turnbull et al. 1988); (11) killed *Bordetella pertussis* (Turnbull et al. 1990); (12) complete Freund's adjuvant (Turnbull et al. 1988); (13) Montanide ISA 51 (purified incomplete Freund's adjuvant) (Ivins, unpublished observations); (14) Quil-A saponin adjuvant (Turnbull et al. 1988); (15) Gasil-23D synthetic silicon dioxide adjuvant (Turnbull et al. 1988); (16) microcapsules (Ivins, unpublished observations); (17) liposomes (Ivins, unpublished observations); (18) β-glucan particles (Adjuvax) (Ivins, unpublished observations); (19) IL-2 (Multikine) (Ivins, unpublished observations); (20) oligonucleotides containing CpG motifs (Ivins, unpublished observations); (21) Matrix M-40

ISCOMS (Ivins, unpublished observations); and (22) polyphosphazene (Ivins, unpublished observations). Many of the above carriers and adjuvants were tested with purified *B. anthracis* PA or rPA in guinea pigs. Some were tested in mice, rabbits, or monkeys in addition to or instead of guinea pigs. Many of the candidate adjuvants or carriers could not be demonstrated to elicit in vaccinated animals either protection or a serological response that was greater than PA combined with an aluminum adjuvant or the US or UK human anthrax vaccine. Adding MPL alone to AVA did not provide a greater protective immune response, but complete Freund's adjuvant, killed *B. pertussis*, or killed *C. ovis* strongly augmented protection when added to the vaccines (Turnbull et al. 1988, 1990). Montanide ISA 51 + PA was not protective in guinea pigs (Ivins, unpublished observations). Interestingly, although this experimental vaccine elicited high ELISA titers, it elicited very low toxin-neutralizing antibody (TNA) titers, suggesting that neutralizing antibodies may be a better predictor of immunity than ELISA titers. Though polyphosphazene + PA has not yet been tested for protective efficacy, it appears in mice to stimulate both anti-PA ELISA and TNA titers better than AVA (Ivins, unpublished observations). When added to AVA, anti-PA titers were also stimulated, but not to the levels seen when the polyphosphazene was added to PA alone. In guinea pigs, oligonucleotides containing CpG motifs appeared to increase the protective efficacy of AVA by a small but definite amount when administered together with the vaccine (Ivins, unpublished observations). T-MDP in SAF-M + PA was more efficacious than AVA in mice but not in guinea pigs (28). Similarly, PA mixed with either QS-21 or MPL was more protective than AVA or PA combined with Alhydrogel in guinea pigs against an aerosol challenge of virulent anthrax spores (Ivins et al. 1995). In monkeys, a single dose of either of those two experimental vaccines (PA with QS-21 or PA with MPL) protected 90%–100% of the animals against an aerosol spore challenge (Ivins et al. 1998). PA mixed with either MPL + CWS or MPL + CWS + TDM was extraordinarily protective against parenteral challenge in guinea pigs (Turnbull 1991; Ivins et al. 1992; McBride et al. 1998). A single dose of the latter protected 95% of animals against a 2,000-LD_{50} challenge of *B. anthracis* spores compared with PA + Alhydrogel, which protected only 25% (Ivins et al. 1992). Similar results were reported with aerosol challenge (McBride et al. 1998). Unfortunately, concern about their potential reactogenicity in humans led to the cessation of investigations involving these two adjuvants. Preliminary experiments in guinea pigs with PA in microcapsules have had disparate results

(Ivins, unpublished observations). The source and size of the microcapsules appear to be quite important in determining the efficacy of the preparation.

5
Summary

In summary, although reliable and safe human anthrax vaccines exist today, they can be improved, particularly by reducing the number of required doses. We anticipate that further advances in the development of new adjuvants and vaccine delivery systems will be made. This knowledge, coupled with the discovery of new potentially protective immunogens aided by the sequencing of the *B. anthracis* genome and by a more complete analysis of the epitopes recognized during infection, may result in a human multicomponent subunit or live vaccine that is highly effective when given in one or two doses.

References

AUERBACH S, WRIGHT GG (1955) Studies on immunity in anthrax. VI. Immunizing activity of protective antigen against various strains of *Bacillus anthracis*. J Immunol 75:129–133

BAIL O (1904) Untersuchungen uber naturliche und kuntliche Milzbrandimmunitat. Centralbl f Bakt 37:270–280

BARNARD JP, FRIEDLANDER AM (1999) Vaccination against anthrax with attenuated recombinant strains of *Bacillus anthracis* that produce protective antigen. Infect Immun 67:562–567

BELTON FC, STRANGE RE (1954) Studies on a protective antigen produced in vitro from *Bacillus anthracis*: medium and methods of production. Br J Exp Pathol 35:144–152

BENSON EL, HUYNH PD, FINKELSTEIN A, COLLIER RJ (1998) Identification of residues lining the anthrax protective antigen channel. Biochemistry 37:3941–3948

BERENDT R, JEMSKI J, JOHNSON-WINEGAR A, IVINS B (1985) The use of toxin components for the immunoprophylaxis of inhalation anthrax. Abstr Ann Meeting Am Soc Microbiol E61:85

BRACHMAN P, FRIEDLANDER AM (1999) Anthrax. In: Plotkin SA, Orenstein WA (eds) Vaccines. W. B. Saunders Philadelphia p. 629–637

BRACHMAN PS, GOLD H, PLOTKIN SA, FEKETY FR, WERRIN M, INGRAHAM NR (1962) Field evaluation of a human anthrax vaccine. Am J Public Health 52:632–645

BROSSIER F, MOCK M, SIRARD J-C (1999) Antigen delivery by attenuated *Bacillus anthracis*: new prospects in veterinary vaccines. J Appl Microbiol 87:298–302

BROSSIER F, WEBER-LEVY M, MOCK M, SIRARD J-C (2000) Role of toxin functional domains in anthrax pathogenesis. Infect Immun 68:1781–1786

Brossier F, Sirard JC, Guidi-Rontani C, Duflot E, Mock M (1999) Functional analysis of the carboxy-terminal domain of *Bacillus anthracis* protective antigen. Infect Immun 67:964–967

Broster MG, Hibbs SE (1990) Protective efficacy of anthrax vaccines against aerosol challenge. Proceedings of the International Workshop on Anthrax, 11–13 April 1989, Winchester, UK Salisbury Med Bull Special suppl No. 68, pp 91–92

Cataldi A, Labruyere E, Mock M (1990) Construction and characterization of a protective antigen-deficient *Bacillus anthracis* strain. Mol Microbiol 4:1111–1117

Chatfield S, Roberts M, Li J, Starns A, Dougan G (1994) The use of live attenuated Salmonella for oral vaccination. Dev Biol Stand 82:35–42

Cohen S, Mendelson I, Altboum Z, Kobiler D, Elhanany E, Bino T, Leitner M, Inbar I, Rosenberg H, Gozes Y, Barak R, Fisher M, Kronman C, Velan B, Shafferman A (2000) Attenuated nontoxigenic and nonencapsulated *Bacillus anthracis* spore vaccines protect against anthrax. Infect Immun 68:4549–4558

Coulson NM, Fulop M, Titball RM (1994) *Bacillus anthracis* protective antigen, expressed in *Salmonella typhimurium* SL3261, affords protection against anthrax spore challenge. Vaccine 12:1395–1401

Cromartie WJ, Watson DW, Bloom WL, Heckly RJ (1947) Studies on infection with *Bacillus anthracis*. II. The immunological and tissue damaging properties of extracts prepared from lesions of *B. anthracis* infection. J Infect Dis 80:14–27

Ezzell JW Jr, Abshire TG (1988) Immunological analysis of cell-associated antigens of *Bacillus anthracis*. Infect Immun 56:349–356

Ezzell JW Jr, Abshire TG (1992) Serum protease cleavage of *Bacillus anthracis* protective antigen. J Gen Microbiol 138:543–549

Farchaus JW, Ribot WJ, Jendrek S, Little SF (1998) Fermentation, purification, and characterization of protective antigen from a recombinant, avirulent strain of *Bacillus anthracis*. Appl Environ Microbiol 64:982–991

Fellows PF, Linscott MK, Ivins BE, Pitt MLM, Rossi CA, Gibbs PH, Friedlander AM (2001) Efficacy of a human anthrax vaccine in guinea pigs, rabbits, and rhesus macaques against challenge by *Bacillus anthracis* isolates of diverse geographical origin. Vaccine (in press)

Fellows PF, Linscott MK, Little SF, Gibbs P, Ivins BE (2000) Anthrax vaccine efficacy in the syrian golden hamster. Abstr Ann Meeting Am Soc Microbiol, Los Angeles CA P. 299 E-28

Friedlander AM, Pittman PR, Parker GW (1999) Anthrax vaccine: evidence for safety and efficacy against inhalational anthrax. JAMA 282:2104–2106

Fubra ES (1966) Nonproteolytic, avirulent *Bacillus anthracis* as a live vaccine. J Bacteriol 91:930–933

Gefen NE, Shustikov VM, Rudneva, OA, Fedyaev SF, Tsimlyansky GT, Golubitsky EA, Lazareva ES (1970) A study of reactogenicity, harmlessness and immunological efficacy of aerosol method of immunization against anthrax in trial on man. Zh Mikrobiol Epidemiol Immunobiol 47:81–85 (In Russian)

Gladstone GP (1946) Immunity to anthrax: protective antigen present in cell-free culture filtrates. Br J Exp Pathol 27:394–418

Gordon RE, Haynes WD, Hor-Nay Pang C (1973) The genus *Bacillus*. U.S. Dep Agric Agric Handb No. 427

Gu M-L, Leppla SH, Klinman DM (1999) Protection against anthrax toxin by vaccination with a DNA plasmid encoding anthrax protective antigen. Vaccine 17:340–344

Gupta P, Waheed SM, Bhatnagar R (1999) Expression and purification of the recombinant protective antigen of *Bacillus anthracis.* Protein Expr Purif 16:369–376

Gupta RK, Siber GR (1995) Adjuvants for human vaccines-current status, problems and future prospects. Vaccine 13:1263–1276

Hambleton P, Carman JA, Turnbull PCB (1984) Anthrax: the disease in relation to vaccines. Vaccine 2:125–132

Hambleton P, Turnbull PCB (1990) Anthrax vaccine development: a continuing story. In: Mizrahi, A (ed) Bacterial Vaccines. Liss, New York, pp 105–122

Hodgson AE (1941) Cutaneous anthrax. Lancet 1:811–813

Iacono-Connors LC, Welkos SL, Ivins BE, Dalrymple JM (1991) Protection against anthrax with recombinant virus-expressed protective antigen in experimental animals. Infect Immun 59:1961–1965

Ivins BE, Ezzell Jr, JW, Jemski J, Hedlund, KW, Ristroph JD, Leppla SH (1986) Immunization studies with attenuated strains of *Bacillus anthracis.* Infect Immun 52:454–458

Ivins BE, Fellows PF, Nelson GO (1994) Efficacy of a standard human anthrax vaccine against *Bacillus anthracis* spore challenge in guinea pigs. Vaccine 12:872–874

Ivins BE, Fellows P, Pitt L, Estep J, Farchaus J, Friedlander A, Gibbs P (1995) Experimental anthrax vaccines: efficacy of adjuvants combined with protective antigen against an aerosol *Bacillus anthracis* spore challenge in guinea pigs. Vaccine 13:1779–1784

Ivins BE, Fellows PF, Pitt MLM, Estep JE, Welkos SL, Worsham PL, Friedlander AM (1996) Efficacy of a standard human anthrax vaccine against *Bacillus anthracis* aerosol spore challenge in rhesus monkeys. Salisbury Med Bull 87: 125–126

Ivins BE, Pitt MLM, Fellows PF, Farchaus JW, Benner GE, Waag DM, Little SF, Anderson JR, Gibbs PH, Friedlander AM (1998) Comparative efficacy of experimental anthrax vaccine candidates against inhalation anthrax in rhesus macaques. Vaccine16:1141–1148

Ivins BE, Welkos SL (1986) Cloning and expression of the *Bacillus anthracis* protective antigen gene in *Bacillus subtilis.* J Bacteriol 54:537–542

Ivins BE, Welkos SL (1988) Recent advances in the development of an improved, human anthrax vaccine. Eur J Epidemiol 4:12–19

Ivins BE, Welkos SL, Knudson GB, Little SF (1990) Immunization against anthrax with aromatic compound-dependent (Aro$^-$) mutants of *Bacillus anthracis* and with recombinant strains of *Bacillus subtilis* that produce anthrax protective antigen. Infect Immun 58:303–308

Ivins BE, Welkos SL, Little SF, Crumrine MH, Nelson GO (1992) Immunization against anthrax with *Bacillus anthracis* protective antigen combined with adjuvants. Infect Immun 60:662–668

Ivins BE, Welkos SL, Little SF, Knudson GB (1990) Cloned protective activity and progress in development of improved anthrax vaccines. Proceedings of the

International Workshop on Anthrax, 11–13 April 1989, Winchester, UK Salisbury Med Bull Special suppl No. 68, pp 86–88

Jackson FC, Wright GG, Armstrong J (1957) Immunization of cattle against experimental anthrax with alum-precipitated protective antigen or spore vaccine. Am J Vet Res 18:771–777

Klein F, DeArmon Jr, IA, Lincoln RE, Mahlandt BG, Fernelius AL (1962) Immunological studies of anthrax. II. Levels of immunity against *Bacillus anthracis* obtained with protective antigen and live vaccine. J Immunol 88:15–19

Leppla SH (1996) Anthrax Toxins in: Moss J, Iglewksi B, Vaughan M, Tu AT (eds) Bacterial toxins and virulence factors in disease. Marcel Dekker Inc P. 543–572

Lincoln RE, Fish DC (1970) Anthrax toxin. In: Montie, TC, Kadis S, Ajl SJ (eds) Microbial Toxins. Academic Press, New York, pp 361–414

Little SF, Ivins BE (1999) Molecular pathogenesis of *Bacillus anthracis* infection. Microbes and Infection 2:131–139

Little SF, Ivins BE, Fellows PF, Friedlander AM (1997) Passive protection studies against *Bacillus anthracis* infection in guinea pigs using monoclonal and polyclonal antibodies. Infect Immun 65:5171–5175

Little SF, Knudson GB (1986) Comparative efficacy of *Bacillus anthracis* live spore vaccine and protective antigen vaccine against anthrax in the guinea pig. Infect Immun 52:509–512

Little SF, Leppla SH, Friedlander AM (1990) Production and characterization of monoclonal antibodies against the lethal factor component of *Bacillus anthracis* lethal toxin. Infect Immun 58:1606–1613

Little SP, Novak JM, Lowe JR, Leppla SH, Singh Y, Klimpel KR, Lidgerding BC, Friedlander AM (1996) Characterization of lethal factor binding and cell receptor binding domains of protective antigen of *Bacillus anthracis* using monoclonal antibodies. Microbiology 142:707–715

Mahlandt BG, Klein F, Lincoln RE, Haines BW, Jones WI, Friedman RH (1966) Immunologic studies of anthrax. IV. Evaluation of the immunogenicity of three components of anthrax toxin. J Immunol 96:727–733

McBride BW, Mogg A, Telfer JL, Lever MS, Miller J, Turnbull PCB, Baillie L (1998) Protective efficacy of a recombinant protective antigen against *Bacillus anthracis* challenge and assessment of immunological markers. Vaccine 16:810–817

Mikesell P, Ivins BE, Ristroph JD, Dreier TM (1983) Evidence for plasmid-mediated toxin production in *Bacillus anthracis*. Infect Immun 38:371–376

Miller J, McBride BW, Manchee RJ, Moore P, Baillie LWJ (1998) Production and purification of recombinant protective antigen and protective efficacy against *Bacillus anthracis*. Lett Appl Microbiol 26:56–60

Novak JM, Stein M-P, Little SF, Leppla SH, Friedlander AM (1992) Functional characterization of protease-treated *Bacillus anthracis* protective antigen. J Biol Chem 267:17186–17193

Oh H-B, Park Y-M, Seong W-K (1998) Expression of *Bacillus anthracis* protective antigen in *Bacillus brevis*. Abstracts of the 3rd International Conference on Anthrax, Plymouth, England, September 7–10, 1998. P. 64.

Pasteur L (1881) De l'attenuation des virus et de leur retour a la virulence. CR Acad Sci Agric Bulg 92:429–435

Petosa C, Collier RJ, Klimpel KR, Leppla SH, Liddington RC (1997) Crystal structure of the anthrax toxin protective antigen. Nature 385:833–838

Pezard C, Berche P, Mock M (1991) Contribution of individual toxin components to virulence of *Bacillus anthracis*. Infect Immun 59:3472–3477

Pezard C, Duflot E, Mock M (1993) Construction of *B. anthracis* mutant strains producing a single toxin component. J Gen Microbiol 139:2459–2463

Pezard C, Weber-Levy M, Sirard J-C, Berche P, Mock M (1995) Protective immunity induced by *Bacillus anthracis* toxin-deficient strains. Infect Immun 63:1369–1372

Pitt MLM, Ivins B, Estep J, Farchaus J, Friedlander AM (1996a) Comparative efficacy of a recombinant protective antigen vaccine against inhalation anthrax in guinea pigs, rabbits, and rhesus monkeys. Abstr Ann Meeting Am Soc Microbiol, Atlanta GA P. 278 E-70

Pitt MLM, Ivins BE, Estep JE, Farchaus J, Friedlander AM (1996b) Comparison of the efficacy of purified protective antigen and MDPH to protect non-human primates from inhalation anthrax. Salisbury Med Bull 87:130

Pitt MLM, Little SF, Ivins BE, Fellows PF, Boles J, Barth J, Hewetson JH, Friedlander, AM (1999) In vitro correlate of immunity in an animal model of inhalational anthrax. J Appl Microbiol 87: 304

Plotkin SL, Plotkin SA (1999) A short history of vaccination. In: Plotkin SA, Orenstein WA (eds) Vaccines. WB Saunders, Philadelphia pp 1–12

Preisz H (1911) Quoted in Anthrax. (1955) In: Wilson GS, Miles AA (eds) Topley and Wilson's Principles of Bacteriology and Immunity. Williams & Wilkins, Baltimore p 1950

Pushko P, Parker M, Ludwig GV, Davis NL, Johnston RE, Smith JF (1997) Replicon-helper systems from attenuated Venezuelan Equine Encephalitis Virus: Expression of heterologous genes in vitro and immunization against heterologous pathogens in vivo. Virology 239:389–401

Puziss M, Manning LC, Lynch LW, Barclay E, Abelow I, Wright GG (1963) Large-scale production of protective antigen of *Bacillus anthracis* anaerobic cultures. Appl Microbiol 11:330–334

Puziss M, Wright GG (1962) Studies on immunity in anthrax. X. Gel-adsorbed protective antigen for immunization of man. J Bacteriol 85:230–236

Salsbery CE (1926) Anthrax aggressin. J Am Vet Med Assn 68:755–772

Sellmann BR, Nassi S, Collier RJ (2001) Point mutations in anthrax protective antigen that block translocation. J Biol Chem 276:8371–8376

Schodel F, Curtiss 3rd R (1995) Salmonella as oral vaccine carriers. Dev Biol Stand 84:245–253

Shlyakhov E, Rubinstein E (1994) Human live anthrax vaccine in the former USSR. Vaccine 12:727–730

Shuylak VP (1970) Epidemiological efficacy of anthrax STI vaccine in Tadjik SSR. Zh Microbiol Epidemiol Immunobiol 47:117–120 (In Russian)

Singh Y, Klimpel KR, Quinn CP, Chaudhary VK, Leppla SH (1991) The carboxyl-terminal end of protective antigen is required for receptor binding and anthrax toxin activity. J Biol Chem 266:15493–15497

Singh Y, Ivins BE, Leppla SH (1998) Study of immunization against anthrax with the purified recombinant protective antigen of *Bacillus anthracis*. Infect Immun 66: 3447–3448

SINGH Y, KLIMPEL KR, GOEL S, SWAIN PK, LEPPLA SH (1999) Oligomerization of anthrax toxin protective antigen and binding of lethal factor during endocytic uptake into mammalian cells. Infect Immun 67:1853–1859

SMITH H, STONER H (1967) Anthrax toxic complex. Fed Proc 26:1554–1557

STANLEY JL, SMITH H (1963) The three factors of anthrax toxin: their immunogenicity and lack of demonstrable enzymatic activity. J Gen Microbiol 31:329–337

STERNE M (1937) Variation in *Bacillus anthracis*. Onderstepoort J Vet Sci Anim Ind 8:271

STERNE M, NICHOL J, LAMBRECHTS NS (1942) The effect of large-scale active immunization against anthrax. J S African Vet Med Assoc 13:53–63

TIGERTT WD (1980) Anthrax. William Smith Greenfield, MD FRCP. Concerning the priority due to him for the production of the first vaccine against anthrax. J Hyg 85:415–420

TURNBULL PCB (1991) Anthrax vaccines: past, present and future. Vaccine 9:533–539

TURNBULL PCB (2000) Current status of immunization against anthrax: old vaccines may be here to stay for a while. Current Opinion in Infectious Diseases 13:113–120

TURNBULL PC, BROSTER, MG, CARMAN JA, MANCHEE RJ, MELLING J (1986) Development of antibodies to protective antigen and lethal factor components of anthrax toxin in humans and guinea pigs and their relevance to protective immunity. Infect Immun 52:356–359

TURNBULL PCB, LEPPLA SH, BROSTER MG, MELLING J (1988) Antibodies to anthrax toxin in humans and guinea pigs and their relevance to protective immunity. Med Microbiol Immunol 177:293–303

TURNBULL PCB, QUINN CP, HEWSON R, STOCKBRIDGE MC, MELLING J (1990) Protection conferred by microbially-supplemented UK and purified PA vaccines. Proceedings of the International Workshop on Anthrax, 11–13 April 1989, Winchester, UK Salisbury Med Bull Special suppl No. 68, pp 89–91

VARUGHESE M, TEIXEIRA AV, LIU S, LEPPLA SH (1999) Identification of a receptor-binding region within domain 4 of the protective antigen component of anthrax toxin. Infect Immun 67:1860–1865

VODKIN M, LEPPLA SH (1983) Cloning of the protective antigen gene of *Bacillus anthracis*. Cell 34:693–696

WATSON DW, CROMARTIE WJ, BLOOM WL, KEGELES G, HECKLY RJ (1947) Studies on infection with *Bacillus anthracis*. III. Chemical and immunological properties of the protective antigen in crude extracts of skin lesions of *B. anthracis*. J Infect Dis 80:28–52

WELKOS S, BECKER D, FRIEDLANDER A, TROTTER R (1990) Pathogenesis and host resistance to *Bacillus anthracis*: a mouse model. Proceedings of the International Workshop on Anthrax, 11–13 April 1989, Winchester, UK Salisbury Med Bull Special suppl No. 68 pp 49–52

WELKOS SL, FRIEDLANDER AM (1988) Comparative safety and efficacy against *Bacillus anthracis* of protective antigen and live vaccines in mice. Microbiol Pathog 5: 127–139

WELKOS SL, VIETRI NJ, GIBBS PH (1993) Non-toxigenic derivatives of the Ames strain of *Bacillus anthracis* are fully virulent for mice: role of plasmid pX02 and chromosome in strain-dependent virulence. Microbial Pathogenesis 14:381–388

Williamson ED, Beedham RJ, Bennett AM, Perkins SD, Miller J, Baillie LW J (1999) Presentation of protective antigen to the mouse immune system: immune sequelae. J Appl Microbiol 87:315–317

Wilson GS, Miles AA (1955) Anthrax. In: Topley and Wilson's Principles of Bacteriology and Immunity. Williams & Wilkins, Baltimore, pp 1938–1954

Worsham PL, Sowers MR (1999) Isolation of an asporogenic (spoOA) protective antigen-producing strain of *Bacillus anthracis*. Can J Microbiol 45:1–8

Wright GG, Green T, Kanode Jr R (1954) Studies on immunity in anthrax. V. Immunizing activity of alum-precipitated protective antigen. J Immunol 73:387–391

Zegers ND, Kluter E, van der Stap H, van Dura E, van Dalen P, Shaw M, Baillie L (1998) Expression of the protective antigen of *Bacillus anthracis* by *Lactobacillus casei*: Towards the development of an oral vaccine against anthrax. J Appl Microbiol 87:309–314

Chapter 4

Structure and Function of Anthrax Toxin

D. B. Lacy, R. J. Collier

D. B. Lacy, R. J. Collier
Department of Microbiology and Molecular Genetics, Harvard Medical School,
Boston, MA 02115, USA, Email: jcollier@hms.harvard.edu.

Abstract. Anthrax toxin is a binary A-B toxin comprised of protective antigen (PA) and two enzymatic moieties, edema factor (EF) and lethal factor (LF). In the presence of a host cell-surface receptor, PA can mediate the delivery of EF and LF from the extracellular milieu into the host cell cytosol to effect toxicity. In this delivery, PA undergoes multiple structural changes – from a monomer to a heptameric prepore to a membrane-spanning heptameric pore. The catalytic factors also undergo dramatic structural changes as they unfold to allow for their translocation across the endosomal membrane and refold to preserve their catalytic activity within the cytosol. In addition to these gross structural changes, the intoxication mechanism depends on the ability of PA to form specific interactions with the host cell receptor, EF, and LF. This chapter presents a review of experiments probing these structural interactions and rearrangements in the hopes of gaining a molecular understanding of toxin action.

1 Introduction

1.1 The Role of Toxins in Virulence

That a toxin might play a role in the pathogenesis of *B. anthracis* was first demonstrated when sterile-filtered serum from infected guinea pigs was shown to cause edema when injected into healthy guinea pigs (Smith et al. 1955). This toxin was resolved into three protein components, and competition experiments indicated that one of the proteins allowed for the action of the other two (Stanley and Smith 1961). These proteins were to be later termed protective antigen (PA), edema factor (EF), and lethal factor (LF). PA, named for its ability to elicit a protective immune response against infection (Gladstone 1946), was required for the activity of both edema and lethal factors but showed no activity when injected alone. The combination of EF and PA produced a skin edema but did not result in death of the animal, whereas LF with PA was lethal but did not produce a skin edema (Stanley and Smith 1961). These early observations were reconfirmed in knock-out experiments in which mutant strains of *B. anthracis* were constructed. LF^- and PA^- mutant strains were not lethal in mice, whereas EF^- strains were lethal but less efficient than wild type (Pezard et al. 1991). Although a synergistic effect for the three proteins administered simultaneously was also observed in the experiments with purified protein (Stanley and Smith 1961), the literature now often refers to two separate toxins: edema toxin (EdTx, PA + EF) and lethal toxin (LeTx, PA + LF) (FRIEDLANDER 1986).

The requirement of three proteins to produce two toxins led to a hypothesis in which EF and LF are enzymes that act on intracellular substrates and require PA for access to the cytosol. It has now been clearly demonstrated that both EdTx and LeTx fall into the class of A-B toxins in that their enzymatic activity ("A" domain) and binding activity ("B" domain) are discrete structures. In the case of EdTx and LeTx, the A and B domains are released from the bacteria as monomeric proteins that combine at the surface of receptor-bearing eukaryotic cells to form toxic complexes. Such toxins have been termed "binary toxins" (GILL 1978).

1.2 General Mechanism

In recent years, an effort to understand the role that EdTx and LeTx play in pathogenesis has resulted in a general model for toxin entry into host cells (LEPPLA et al. 1987). This mechanism (Fig. 1) involves PA binding to

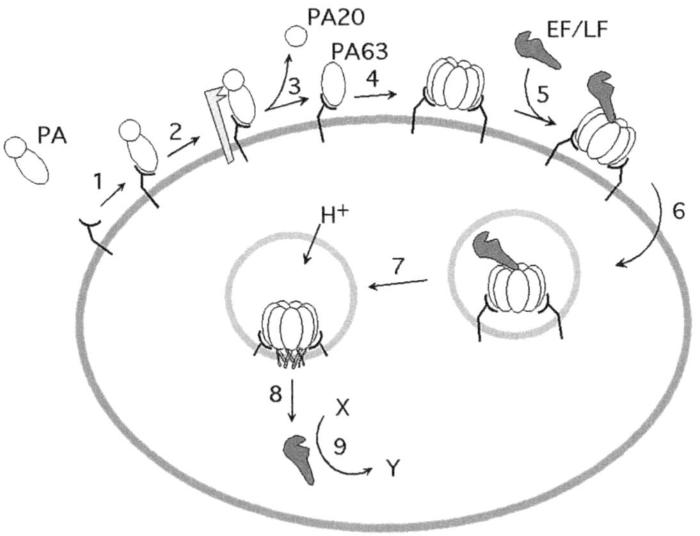

Fig. 1. Steps in anthrax toxin intoxication. PA_{83} binds the extracellular receptor and becomes activated by furin or a furin-like protease. PA_{20} diffuses away while PA_{63} oligomerizes to form a heptamer. EF and LF bind the heptamer and become internalized by receptor-mediated endocytosis. Acidification of the endosome leads to pore formation and translocation of the "A" moiety into the cytosol, where catalysis occurs

a cell surface receptor and its proteolytic activation. This allows for oligomerization and binding of the catalytic factor(s). It is thought that the toxin complex is internalized by receptor-mediated endocytosis and is exposed to the acidic pH of the endosome. This change in pH is believed to trigger both pore formation and translocation of the catalytic factor(s) across the endosomal membrane into the cytosol. The enzymatic A moiety is then free to act on its cytosolic target, thus triggering the cascade of events that results in the disease symptoms of anthrax. This review presents a summary of the structural and functional experiments geared toward obtaining a molecular understanding of this intoxication mechanism.

2 PA Structure

The genes for PA, EF, and LF are all located on the pXO1 plasmid (Mikesell et al. 1983). Each gene has been cloned (Vodkin and Leppla 1983; Robertson and Leppla 1986; Mock et al. 1988; Tippetts and Robertson 1988) and sequenced (Robertson et al. 1988; Welkos et al. 1988; Bragg and Robertson 1989), and each encodes a secreted protein. It is notable that PA, EF, and LF do not contain any cysteine residues, a fact that may be relevant for their activity in oxidizing environments (Hanna et al. 1994).

The mature PA protein is 735 amino acids (83 kDa). It shares sequence homology with a family of binary ADP-ribosyltransferase toxins, aligning to the B moieties of *Clostridium botulinum* C2 (33% identity), *Clostridium difficile* cdt (35% identity), *Clostridium perfringens* iota-toxin-1b (34% identity), *Clostridium spiroforme* Sb (33% identity), and the *Bacillus cereus* vegetative insecticidal protein (VIP1) (27% identity). A number of biophysical techniques aimed at elucidating secondary, tertiary, and quaternary structures have been applied to PA. Of particular note have been the crystallographic analyses performed by Liddington and co-workers. The crystal structure of monomeric PA, determined at 2.1 Å, revealed the presence of four structural domains within the molecule (Fig. 2A) (Petosa et al. 1997). Domain 1 (residues 1–249) primarily adopts a β-sandwich fold with a jelly-roll topology. Because it contains the proteolytic activation site, it is divided into two subdomains, 1a, corresponding to the 20-kDa fragment removed with cleavage, and 1b, which is part of the larger, 63-kDa fragment. Subdomain 1b contains two structural calcium ions coordinated through a modified EF-hand motif. Domain 2 (residues 250–487)

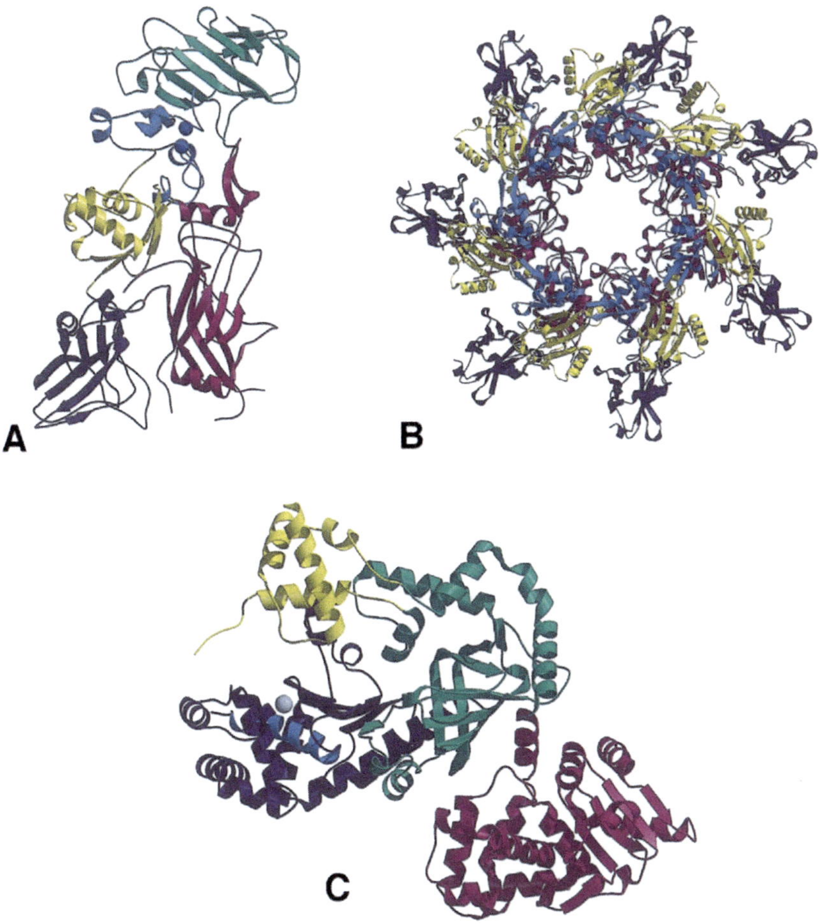

Fig. 2 A–C. Crystallographic structures of PA_{83}, $(PA_{63})_7$, and LF. **A** PA_{83} with domain 1a in *green*, domain 1b and the two calcium ions in *blue*, domain 2 in *magenta*, domain 3 in *yellow*, and domain 4 in *purple*. **B** A SDS-resistant PA_{63} heptamer that may represent a prepore conformation shown in an axial view and colored as in **A**. **C** LF with LFn colored in *magenta*, the ADP-ribosyltransferase fold colored in *green*, the repeat region colored in *yellow*, and the C-terminal zinc protease domain colored in *purple*. The HEXXH helix coordinating the catalytic zinc (*gray sphere*) is highlighted in *blue*

is a β-barrel core with large loops, including a flexible loop between $2\beta_2$ and $2\beta_3$ that has been implicated in pore formation. Domain 3 is the smallest of the four domains and consists of residues 488–594. It has a four-stranded mixed β-sheet, four small helices, and a fold similar to that of ferredoxins and domain A of toxic-shock-syndrome-toxin-1 (Petosa et al. 1997). Efforts to identify its function point to a role in oligomerization (Mogridge et al. 2001). Domain 4 (595–735) comprises the receptor binding domain. It is a β-sandwich with an immunoglobin-like fold and has limited contact with the other three structural domains.

After proteolytic cleavage, subdomain 1a (PA_{20}) is thought to diffuse away from the receptor bound PA_{63} fragment. The latter fragment is capable of spontaneously oligomerizing in solution to form a heptamer, $(PA_{63})_7$, and there is evidence that a similar form generates the pore and translocates EF and LF to the cytosol. A heptameric species of PA_{63} has been crystallized and its structure solved at 4.5 Å (Fig. 2B), revealing a ring-shaped oligomer with a negatively charged lumen (Petosa et al. 1997). This oligomer may represent a pore precursor or prepore. Domain 2 lines the lumen of this species and mediates the majority of the intermonomer contacts. The structure reveals a channel whose average diameter is 35 Å and can narrow to as small as 20 Å.

3 Binding the Cell Surface Receptor

3.1 Characteristics of the Receptor

In general, the specific binding of a toxin to a cell surface receptor is a key determinant of host cell sensitivity and intoxication efficiency (Eidels et al. 1983). Although the receptor for anthrax toxin remains unidentified, experiments on the Chinese hamster ovary cell line CHO-K1 indicate that the receptor is at least partially proteinaceous and that the interaction between PA and the receptor is highly specific and saturable (Escuyer and Collier 1991). Efforts to identify the receptor with chemical crosslinking of ^{125}I-PA to cells yielded a 170-kDa band on a SDS-polyacrylamide gel. This implies linkage of PA to a protein of roughly 90 kDa (Escuyer and Collier 1991).

The receptor seems ubiquitous inasmuch as a varied array of cell types respond to EdTx. Cellular responses to EdTx can be followed through cell shape changes, cAMP concentrations, or the cAMP-regulated Cl^- secretion induced by EF entry (LEPPLA 1982b; BEAUREGARD et al. 1999). With the latter technique, the receptor was found to be on the basolateral side of polarized epithelial cells but not on the apical side (BEAUREGARD et al. 1999). Furthermore, unlike cholera toxin receptors, the receptor does not fractionate with the insoluble caveola-like membranes.

3.2
Characteristics of the PA Receptor-Binding Domain

The idea that domain 4 contains the receptor-binding function is directly supported by the observation that a fragment of PA corresponding to residues 663–735 is able to compete with full-length PA for binding (NOSKOV et al. 1996). Furthermore, two monoclonal antibodies that recognize the region between residues 671 and 721 have been shown to block PA binding to its receptor (LITTLE et al. 1988, 1996). In an effort to determine the role of the extreme C-terminus of PA in binding, an assay measuring competition between intact ^{125}I-PA and PA proteins truncated by 3, 5, 7, 12, or 14 amino acids was performed (SINGH et al. 1991). Deletions of 3, 5, or 7 amino acids resulted in a 2- to 10-fold reduction in cell binding activity, whereas the 12- and 14-residue deletions completely eliminated it. These data indicate that the integrity of the C-terminal 14 residues is required for binding of PA to the cell receptor, either through direct interactions or by maintaining a structural scaffold. The antibody mapping experiments (LITTLE et al. 1988, 1996) and more recent experiments substituting the C-terminal 3–5 residues with nonnative amino acids supports the latter hypothesis (VARUGHESE et al. 1999). Two solvent-exposed loops of domain 4 (704–723 and 679–693) have been tested for possible interactions with the receptor. Deletion of residues 711–721 and 705–722 yielded PA molecules that were 10 times less active than wild type (BROSSIER et al. 1999). However, alanine scanning mutagenesis indicated that replacement of native amino acids in the 704–723 loop had no effect on binding whereas replacement of residues in or near the 679–693 loop had a major effect, indicating a direct role of the latter in the interaction with the receptor (VARUGHESE et al. 1999).

Finally, it is interesting to note that the sequence homology observed between PA and the ADP-ribosyltransferase binary toxins does not extend to domain 4 (PETOSA et al. 1997). This could indicate different receptor specificities of the toxins.

4
Activation by Proteolysis

The cleavage of receptor-bound PA_{83} to yield PA_{63} is a critical step in intoxication because loss of PA_{20} is thought to expose a site for the binding of EF and/or LF and to relieve steric hinderances that block oligomerization (Petosa et al. 1997). The cleavage can be achieved in vitro with low concentrations of trypsin. Trypsin cleavage at Arg167 was deduced by N-terminal sequencing, and it was hypothesized that the in vivo cleavage would occur at or near the same site. To test this, a PA variant with residues 163–168 deleted was constructed. This molecule was not cleaved by trypsin or the in vivo protease and was completely nontoxic on cells and in rats when administered with LF (Singh et al. 1989). This site in PA is comprised of four basic residues: Arg^{164}-Lys^{165}-Lys^{166}-Arg^{167}. Evidence that the ubiquitously expressed endoprotease furin cleaved a consensus site of Arg-X-Lys/Arg-Arg led to the hypothesis that furin might cleave PA (Molloy et al. 1992). In fact, cleavage of PA by furin was observed in vitro (Molloy et al. 1992), and furin inhibitors blocked cleavage of receptor-bound PA on cells (Klimpel et al. 1992). Although furin has been primarily localized to the Golgi apparatus by immunochemical methods (Bresnahan et al. 1990), at least a small amount of furin seems to be present on the cell surface (Klimpel et al. 1992).

The experiments with furin do not exclude the possibility that other proteases could be acting at the cell surface to activate PA. Furin-deficient CHO cells, selected by chemical mutagenesis, were shown to be sensitive to PA and a LF-*Pseudomonas* exotoxin A fusion, implying the presence of additional cellular proteases (Gordon et al. 1995). Other members of the furin protease family have been shown to cleave PA; they include PC1 (Friedman et al. 1995) and PACE4 (Gordon et al. 1997).

5
Oligomerization

Evidence that PA forms ring-shaped heptamers after proteolytic activation was initially obtained by electron microscopy of purified PA_{63} (Milne et al. 1994). Such a structure correlates with the property of purified PA_{63} being able to form ion-conductive pores (channels) in model membranes and the plasma membrane of receptor-bearing cells (Blaustein et al. 1989; Koehler and Collier 1991; Milne and Collier 1993). Studies in model membranes have shown that single channels are indeed oligomeric (BENSON et al. 1998). Finally, recent evidence from the characterization of dominant negative mutant forms of PA is consistent with the hypothesis that PA-mediated translocation involves an obligatory heptameric intermediate (SELLMAN et al. 2001).

The crystal structure of the heptameric prepore indicates that a number of residues in domain 2 mediate monomer-monomer interactions within the heptamer (PETOSA et al. 1997). However, mutation of a single one of these residues can have a profound effect on the formation and/or stability of the heptamer. For example, the PA483QA mutant protein was less efficient both in forming heptamer and in translocating ^{35}S-labeled LFn (MOGRIDGE et al. 2001). Residues involved in heptamerization have also been identified in domain 3. Mutation at the tip of a domain 3 loop, PA512DA, results in a protein severely deficient in its ability to oligomerize and form channels (MOGRIDGE et al. 2001).

6
EF/LF Binding to PA

EF and LF share sequence homology in the N-terminal 250 residues but differ dramatically in the C-terminus. This observation led to the hypothesis that the N-terminal domain mediates the common binding and internalization functions whereas the catalytic function is carried out by the C-terminal domains (BRAGG and ROBERTSON 1989). This is supported in LF by in-frame insertion mutagenesis experiments showing that, whereas insertions in the N-terminal third of LF eliminated both toxicity and binding to PA, insertions in the C-terminal third eliminated toxicity without affecting PA binding (QUINN et al. 1991). Similarly in EF, binding of two mABs whose antigenic sites mapped within residues 1–156 of EF was found to block binding of EF to PA (LITTLE et al. 1994).

In an effort to identify the minimal LF domain required for PA binding and internalization, several N-terminal LF sequences were fused to the ADP-ribosyltransferase domain of *Pseudomonas* exotoxin A and tested for toxicity (ARORA and LEPPLA 1993). By protein synthesis inhibition assay in CHO cells, the fusion protein containing LF residues 1–254 (LFn) was toxic when administered with PA whereas a fusion with residues 1–198 was inactive. This experiment further proves that the PA binding domain lies within residues 1–254 of LF and provides a minimal protein for the delivery of heterologous peptides and proteins with anthrax toxin.

Attempts to identify residues involved directly in the binding interactions have focused on both the catalytic factors and PA. LF modification with diethyl pyrocarbonate (DEPC) resulted in the loss of binding and toxicity. Because DEPC primarily modifies histidine residues, the nine histidine residues of LFn were then tested individually by site-directed mutagenesis. A His35Gly mutation resulted in a 20-fold drop in toxicity (ARORA 1997). In experiments designed to probe the interactions with antibodies, four mAbs that inhibited LF binding to cell-bound PA were mapped to two distinct antigenic sites of PA: 168–314 and 581–601. This experiment suggests that LF may interact with two different sites on PA (LITTLE et al. 1996).

A quantitative analysis of the binding affinity of EF for $(PA_{63})_7$ with surface plasmon resonance revealed a k_{on} of ~3×10^5 M^{-1} s^{-1}, a k_{off} of $(3–5) \times 10^{-4}$ s^{-1}, and a calculated K_d of $(1–2) \times 10^{-9}$ M (ELLIOTT et al. 2000). A similar K_d (7×10^{-10} M) was obtained from measurements of radiolabeled EF to receptor-bound PA_{63} on cells, indicating that the receptor does not play a significant role in the interaction between EF and PA_{63}. Similar results were obtained with LF and LFn bound to PA_{63}.

7
Receptor-Mediated Endocytosis

BEAUREGARD et al. (BEAUREGARD et al. 2000) have reported data indicating that oligomerization triggers receptor-mediated endocytosis of receptor-bound PA_{63}. This conclusion was based on the findings that a furin-resistant form of PA remained at the cell surface for prolonged periods and that excess PA_{20} inhibited clearance of PA_{63}, presumably by blocking oligomerization. PA was converted on the cell surface to a pronase-resistant form characteristic of oligomeric PA_{63} in solution, a fact that further implicated oligomerization as the triggering event for endocytosis.

An in vitro assay that explored the sensitivity of macrophages to LeTx provided the first experimental evidence that the toxin requires passage through an acidic endocytic vesicle (FRIEDLANDER 1986). Incubation of cells with lysomotropic amines or monensin eliminated the intracellular proton gradients and resulted in protection from LeTx. Analogous experiments using inhibitors of endosome acidification (ammonium chloride or chloroquine) or an inhibitor of endocytosis (cytochalasin D) were performed for EdTx (GORDON et al. 1988). Finally, inhibitors of the vacuolar ATPase proton pump (bafilomycin and concanamycin A) were shown to prevent LeTx toxicity in macrophages (MENARD et al. 1996). All experiments support the hypothesis that the toxin reaches the cytosol via the endosome. The required exposure to acidic pH is thought to be due to a pH-dependent trigger for pore formation and translocation.

8
Pore Formation

The PA_{63} fragment, now known to form a heptamer, was first shown to form channels in planar phospholipid bilayers (BLAUSTEIN et al. 1989). The channels were cation selective and pH- and voltage dependent. Since then, the channel forming properties of PA_{63} have also been observed in liposomes and mammalian cells (KOEHLER and COLLIER 1991; MILNE and COLLIER 1993). Proteolysis and mutagenesis experiments implicated residues 302–325 of domain 2 in the insertion process (NOVAK et al. 1992; SINGH et al. 1994). Proteolysis in this chymotrypsin-sensitive loop was shown to have no effect on receptor binding, LF binding, or internalization, but did result in a loss of toxicity (NOVAK et al. 1992). Mutagenesis at the actual site of cleavage specifically implicated the importance of residues Phe^{313} and Phe^{314} in the intoxication of cells (SINGH et al. 1994) and a PA mutant deleted for residues Phe^{313}-Phe^{314}-Asp^{315} did not interact with liposomes containing a photoactivatable lipid (WANG et al. 1998).

Potential clues as to how the PA_{63} heptamer might insert into membranes came from structural studies on the α-hemolysin from *Staphylococcal aureus*. This is also a pore-forming bacterial toxin that forms heptamers. Its crystal structure, which was solved in detergent to trigger the membrane-spanning conformation (Fig. 3; SONG et al. 1996), revealed a heptamer in which each monomer contributes a β-hairpin to form a 14-stranded β-barrel spanning the membrane. The β-hairpin contains alternating hydrophilic and hydrophobic residues as does the chymotrypsin-sensitive loop in PA.

The crystal structures of PA_{83} and the $(PA_{63})_7$ prepore did not reveal electron density for the 302–325 loop, implying that it is disordered before insertion in the membrane (PETOSA et al. 1997). However, the location of the residues preceding this sequence imply that the loop projects out from domain 2 away from the heptamer. A model for the conformational change required for insertion was based on the structure. In this model, the Greek-key motif (formed by 4 β-strands of domain 2) unfolds and "peels" away from the main body of the heptamer to allow the loop to insert and span the membrane (Fig. 4). Of the nine histidines within PA_{63}, five are located within the Greek-key motif and could become protonated with the

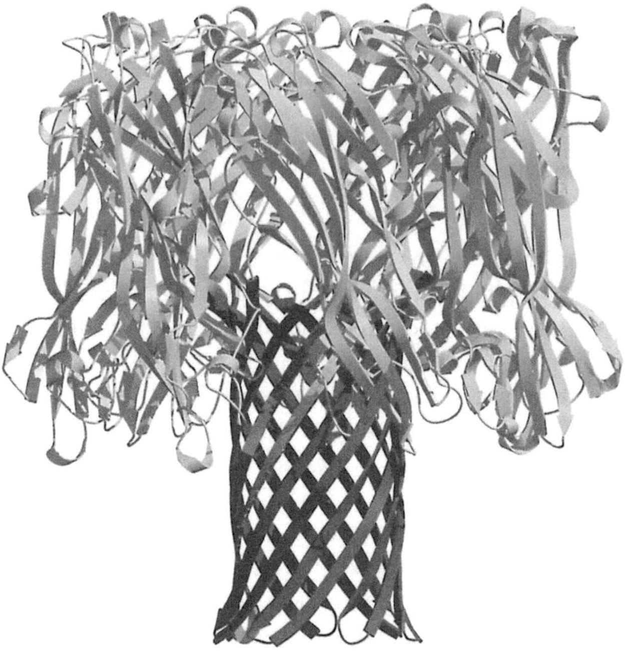

Fig. 3. Crystallographic structure of *S. aureus* α-hemolysin. The 7 monomers oligomerize to form a 14-stranded β-barrel (*dark gray*) spanning the membrane

pH change of the endosome. Two of the histidines (His^{304} and His^{310}) are located within the insertion loop and are thought not to be involved in triggering the insertion (Miller et al. 1999). Another two of these five histidines (His^{263} and His^{299}) are located within a pocket of buried polar residues at the location where the loop joins the top of the Greek-key motif. Their protonation could lead to local instability and unfolding. The final histidine (His^{336}) is located in a loop at the base of the Greek-key motif. This loop was ordered in crystals grown at pH 7.5 but disordered at pH 6.0 and, therefore, may represent a region of the structure that will change with membrane insertion (Petosa et al. 1997).

The results of channel conductance experiments using a Cys-reactive probe support the structural model in which the 302–325 loop inserts to form a 14-stranded β-barrel spanning the membrane (Benson et al. 1998). Twenty-four consecutive amino acids of the loop were individually mutated to cysteine. After tryptic activation and pore formation in planar phospholipid bilayers, the mutant proteins were labeled with methanethiosul-

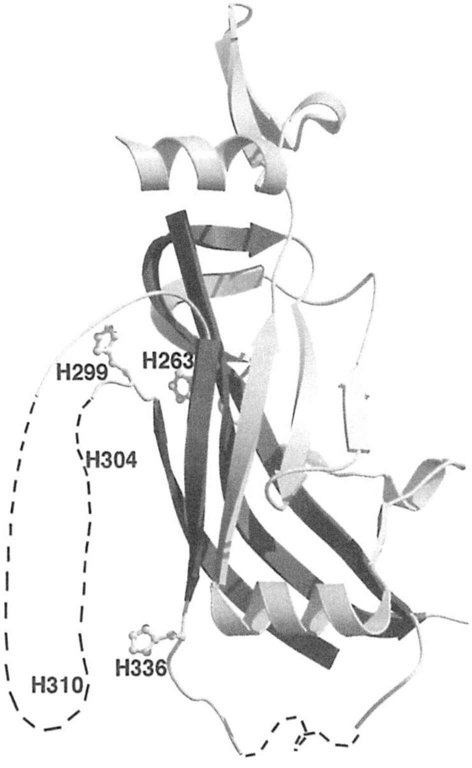

Fig. 4. Domain 2 of PA. The *dotted lines* represent the 302–325 insertion loop and the loop that was disordered at pH 6.0. Unfolding of 2 β-strands from the Greek-key motif (*dark gray*) is thought to allow the 302–325 loop to span the membrane

fonate ethyltrimethylammonium (MTS-ET), a positively charged, membrane-impermeant probe, added to the *trans* compartment of the apparatus. The experimental premise was that the additional positive charge would reduce the channel conductance observed in bilayers when the probe was located within the ion-conducting channel. Results from these experiments showed alternating current reduction over the stretches 302–311 and 316–325, consistent with the alternating polar and apolar residues that would be present on β-strands exposed to both a water-filled lumen and a lipid bilayer.

The PA_{63} heptamer appears to exist in multiple conformations. Our current working model is that PA_{63} oligomerization on cells proceeds through a SDS-sensitive and pronase-resistant stage. Exposure of receptor-bound

SDS-sensitive heptamer to low pH (ca. pH 5) presumably converts it to an SDS-resistant form, as observed by Milne et al. (Milne et al. 1994). This transition includes structural changes in both the $2\beta2-2\beta3$ loop and other regions of PA_{63} as evidenced by the conversion of a PA_{63} mutant with a deleted $2\beta2-2\beta3$ loop to an SDS-resistant heptamer (Miller et al. 1999). This mutant could bind receptor and EF/LF but was unable to form pores or translocate protein.

The crystallographic analysis suggested the unfolding of the Greek-key motif in domain 2 and the movement of domain 4 to accommodate the insertion of the $2\beta2-2\beta3$ loop (Petosa et al. 1997; Miller et al. 1999). A more recent biochemical analysis of the transformation indicates that additional structural changes are occurring in the lumen of the heptamer cap (Sellman et al. 2001). Lys^{397} and Asp^{425} are solvent-exposed residues in the lumen of the prepore. Although distant from the $2\beta2-2\beta3$ loop, mutation of these residues to alanine results in SDS-sensitive heptamers that do not become SDS resistant, form channels, or translocate protein. K397D is also completely inactive, K397Q is inactive but does form SDS-resistant heptamers, whereas K397R is almost fully active. This suggests a structural rearrangement in this site and a requirement for a positive charge in the transition of prepore to pore. Similar to the K397Q mutation, a F427A mutation was nonfunctional but retained the ability to form SDS-resistant oligomers.

9 Translocation

9.1 Translocation Models

It is unknown whether pore formation is a prerequisite or a consequence of translocation. Although the functions have been correlated empirically in that all mutants deficient in translocation are also unable to form pores, the mechanistic relationship has not been proven. In the initial planar lipid bilayer experiments, channel conductance was not observed with EF, LF, PA_{83}, or PA_{20} (Blaustein et al. 1989). This led to the proposal that EF and LF are passively translocated across the endosomal membrane via the PA_{63} channel (Koehler and Collier 1991; Arora and Leppla 1993). However, experiments using radioactive phospholipid probes have shown that both EF and LF (in addition to PA_{83} and PA_{63}) insert into bilayers in a pH-dependent manner and, at sufficiently low pH, can destabilize the membrane (KOCHI et al. 1994). This raises the possibility that the catalytic subunits have an active role in their translocation and that they could, for example, cross the membrane at the PA_{63}-lipid interface. The A moieties probably cannot translocate the membrane independent of PA_{63}, as the experiments do indicate that the pH profiles for membrane destabilization and translocation in cells are characteristic of PA (KOCHI et al. 1994). Therefore, because the evidence supports formation of the heptamer prepore on the cell surface and pH-induced $(PA_{63})_7$ insertion within the endosome, it seems plausible that pore formation precedes or occurs simultaneously with translocation. Questions such as whether the insertion drives translocation, whether the catalytic factors have an active role in the process, and whether the translocation occurs through the pore lumen or at the protein-lipid interface remain to be answered.

9.2
Catalytic Factor Unfolding

Regardless of whether the A moiety translocates via the pore or via the protein-lipid interface, it seems likely that the ~90-kDa catalytic factors will have to unfold and then refold in the cytoplasm. Experiments showing that LF underwent hydrogen/deuterium exchange faster in the presence of liposomes were suggestive of unfolding (WANG et al. 1996). More direct evidence came from experiments done in an in vivo translocation assay (WESCHE et al. 1998). LFn was fused to the catalytic domain of diphtheria toxin (DTA) and dihydrofolate reductase (DHFR) to create the constructs LFn-DTA and LFn-DHFR. Translocation of LFn-DTA was blocked by the introduction of an artificial disulfide in DTA or the presence of the DTA ligand adenine. The translocation of LFn-DHFR was also blocked in the presence of its ligand, methotrexate. The structural constraints imposed by the disulfide or ligand suggest that at least partial unfolding is required for translocation.

9.3
Translocation of Heterologous Proteins

As implied by the LFn-DTA experiments, PA has been shown to be able to translocate heterologous proteins into the cytosol. Proteins can be fused to either the N- or C-terminus of LFn, implying that the N-terminus of LFn does not have to be free (ARORA and LEPPLA 1994). In fact, LFn, or binding to the EF/LF binding site on PA, is not absolutely required, as polycationic peptides were capable of delivering DTA to the cytosol via PA (Blanke et al. 1996). One potential application of PA's ability to deliver heterologous proteins is in the construction of vaccines designed to elicit a cytotoxic T lymphocyte (CTL) response (Ballard et al. 1996). A review outlining the use of bacterial toxins in this delivery indicates that anthrax toxin is the most promising of the toxins, given its efficiency of translocation and ability to transfer large proteins (Goletz et al. 1997).

10
Edema Factor

10.1
EF Is an Adenylate Cyclase

The similarity between the edematous response from EdTx and that from cholera toxin (CT) led to the hypothesis that EF, like CT, acts by elevating cAMP (Leppla 1982a). A difference in kinetics of cAMP formation suggested that unlike CT, which acts by modifying an adenylate cyclase, EF actually is an adenylate cyclase (AC). Furthermore, the activity was shown to be calmodulin dependent, as the cell lysate required for activity could be replaced with purified calmodulin.

Bordetella pertussis also produces a calmodulin-dependent adenylate cyclase. The genes encoding these toxins have very different GC contents but were shown to have three highly conserved domains of amino acid sequence (Robertson 1988). In EF these domains correspond to residues 303–339, 454–466, and 534–557. The first of these domains, 303–339, is comprised of a conserved 24-amino acid peptide that is thought to be part of the ATP binding site and has similarity to eukaryotic ACs (Escuyer et al. 1988; Goyard et al. 1989). In fact, mAbs raised against residues 309–325 were used to identify a new class of mammalian ACs (Orlando et al. 1992). Mammalian ACs are integral membrane proteins that act as heterodimers to play a critical role in signaling. It is unclear whether the bacterial ACs represent convergent or divergent evolution. The observation that EF interaction with lipids is pH independent raised the interesting suggestion that EF could remain tethered to the membrane once reaching the cytosol, perhaps mimicking the eukaryotic AC function (Wang et al. 1997). In support of this hypothesis, a selective permeabilization assay showed association of radioactive EF with vesicle membranes after translocation (Guidi-Rontani et al. 2000).

10.2
EF Structure

EF is composed of at least three functionally distinct domains. As in LF, removing the N-terminal 261 residues of EF has no effect on catalytic activity, consistent with this domain being involved in PA binding but not catalysis (LABRUYERE et al. 1990). The catalytic activity is confined to the remaining portion of the molecule and can be separated into substrate- and calmodulin-binding subdomains. Site-directed mutagenesis has shown the importance of the 303–339 sequence in catalysis. In particular, Lys^{313} seems to ensure tight binding of the nucleotide substrate (XIA and STORM 1990; LABRUYERE et al. 1991). Histidines can act as general bases in cyclization and have been examined for the *B. pertussis* AC (MUNIER et al. 1992). Of the nine His residues in *B. pertussis* AC, three are conserved with EF. His^{63}, which by homology should be equivalent to His^{318} of EF, is not essential for binding nucleotides but has a profound impact on the kinetics of catalysis. The final subdomain is involved in binding calmodulin. A peptide corresponding to residues 499–532 of EF can bind calmodulin in a calcium-dependent manner with wild-type affinity (MUNIER et al. 1993). However, photoaffinity labeling of EF with radioactive calmodulin followed by sequential chemical cleavage indicates that the C-terminal 150 residues are involved in calmodulin binding (LABRUYERE et al. 1990).

The N-terminal domain of EF is likely to have structural homology to that of LF, whereas the C-terminal subdomains could differ dramatically given the divergent sequence and function. A secondary structure analysis of the C-terminal 541 residues of EF with Fourier transform infrared spectroscopy and circular dichroism indicates that the secondary structure is mainly β-strand (LABRUYERE et al. 1991).

11
Lethal Factor

11.1
LF Is a Zinc Endoprotease

The first clue to the function of LF came from the identification of the HEXXH zinc metalloprotease consensus sequence in residues 686–690 (KLIMPEL et al. 1994). Mutation of His^{686}, Glu^{687}, or His ^{690} inactivated LF and led to a decreased binding of ^{65}Zn in the case of the His mutations.

These data, along with the observation of inhibition with bestatin and captopril, known zinc protease inhibitors, led to the proposal that LF is a zinc protease. Other bacterial zinc proteases include the clostridial neurotoxins tetanus and botulinum neurotoxin. LF does not share significant sequence homology with these toxins.

Even after deducing the activity of LF, the in vivo substrate remained an unknown until recently. By two different techniques, LF was shown to cleave the N-terminus of Mek1 and Mek2, mitogen-activated protein kinase (MAPK) kinases (MAPKKs) (DUESBERY et al. 1998; VITALE et al. 1998). The result is that the MAPKs ERK1 and ERK2, which dock to the N-terminus of MAPKKs, become phosphoryated (VITALE et al. 1998). The cascade of events that follows remains unclear, but some evidence does suggest a role of the proteasome, perhaps in the degradation of molecules required for macrophage homeostasis (TANG and LEPPLA 1999).

11.2 LF Structure

The three-dimensional structure of LF (Fig. 2C) has recently been solved to 2.3 Å (R. Liddington, personal communication.) The structure spans residues 28–777 and reveals a clear structural distinction between the PA-binding N-terminus (LFn) and the catalytic C-terminus. The N-terminal domain (27–262), corresponding to LFn, is α-helical except for 6 β-strands forming a 4-stranded and a 2-stranded β-sheet on one face of the molecule. The C-terminus can be divided into two distinct domains. The first (263–550) is formed by nine successive α-helices followed by a β-sheet core in which a 5-stranded mixed β-sheet with an additional α-helix packs perpendicular to a 3-stranded antiparallel β-sheet. The final domain (551–777) contains the zinc protease active site. It is predominantly α-helical, with the exception of a 4-stranded β-sheet, characteristic of other zinc proteases, which buttresses the HEXXH helix.

The active site lies in a cleft formed by the two C-terminal domains. The structure supports the hypothesis that Glu^{687} acts as a ligand for the catalytic water whereas residues His^{686} and His^{690} directly coordinate the zinc. It identifies Glu^{735} as the fourth ligand and also points to a possible role for Tyr^{728} in catalysis or substrate recognition. The position of Tyr^{728} in LF is identical to the position of Tyr^{365} in the structure of botulinum neurotoxin type A (BoNT/A) (LACY et al. 1998). This tyrosine is noteworthy because of its proximity to the zinc (3.3 Å in LF) and because of the fact that it is strictly conserved among eight clostridial neurotoxin sequences and now LF.

A comparison of the structural fold of the LF zinc protease domain to other zinc proteases, including BoNT/A, indicates only weak homology, limited to the HEXXH helix and the neighboring 4-stranded β-sheet. Surprisingly, however, the fold is highly homologous to that of LFn. The domains share an identical topology and overlay with a root mean square deviation (rmsd) of 2.0 Å for 100 C-α atoms. There is 26% sequence identity between the two domains, but the "HEXXH helix" residues differ such that LFn does not bind zinc. (In LFn the sequence in this helix is YEIGK as opposed to HEFGH in the C-terminal zinc protease domain.)

The only structural similarity between LF and other proteins is a significant homology between the C-terminal domain 263–550 and the ADP-ribosyltransferase from the *B. cereus* vegetative insecticidal protein toxin VIP2. The structures align with an rmsd of 2.2 Å for 184 C-αatoms and differ only in a structural deviation in LF residues 300–386. The residues between 300 and 386 form a helical protrusion from the ADP-ribosyltransferase fold that forms the boundary of the zinc protease cleft. This stretch of amino acids was noted earlier for its primary sequence, which contains a series of four imperfect 19-amino acid repeats. A deletion of the first of these four repeats (residues 308–326) rendered the protein nontoxic (ARORA and LEPPLA 1993) and indicates that, although structurally distinct from the rest of the molecule, this domain may play a role in substrate specificity and/or catalysis.

Furthermore, the structural homology to an ADP-ribosylating toxin could have exciting implications for the evolution of LeTx. Given the sequence homology of PA with the B moieties of the ADP-ribosyltransferase binary toxins and the structural homology between LF and VIP2, the two A moieties for which there are structures, it is intriguing to consider that LeTx arose through divergent evolution. The addition of a zinc protease fold at the beginning and end of the ADP-ribosyltransferase fold, along with the insertion of a series of sequence repeats, could result in a new toxin where the ADP-ribosylation activity is no longer required. Alternatively, LeTx may have once existed in a simpler form, with the addition of the ADP-ribosyltransferase domain representing a later insertion.

Acknowledgements. We thank Jeremy Mogridge and Michael Mourez for critical comments on the manuscript and Robert Liddington for providing the LF coordinates before publication.

References

Arora N (1997) Site directed mutagenesis of histidine residues in anthrax toxin lethal factor binding domain reduces toxicity. Mol Cell Biochem 177:7–14

Arora N, Leppla SH (1993) Residues 1–254 of anthrax toxin lethal factor are sufficient to cause cellular uptake of fused polypeptides. J Biol Chem 268:3334–41

Arora N, Leppla SH (1994) Fusions of anthrax toxin lethal factor with shiga toxin and diphtheria toxin enzymatic domains are toxic to mammalian cells. Infect Immun 62:4955–61

Ballard JD, Collier RJ, Starnbach MN (1996) Anthrax toxin-mediated delivery of a cytotoxic T-cell epitope in vivo. Proc Natl Acad Sci USA 93:12531–4

Beauregard KE, Collier RJ, Swanson JA (2000) Proteolytic activation of receptor-bound anthrax protective antigen on macrophages promotes its internalization. Cell Microbiol 2:251–258

Beauregard KE, Wimer-Mackin S, Collier RJ, Lencer WI (1999) Anthrax toxin entry into polarized epithelial cells. Infect Immun 67:3026–30

Benson EL, Huynh PD, Finkelstein A, Collier RJ (1998) Identification of residues lining the anthrax protective antigen channel. Biochemistry 37:3941–8

Blanke SR, Milne JC, Benson EL, Collier RJ (1996) Fused polycationic peptide mediates delivery of diphtheria toxin A chain to the cytosol in the presence of anthrax protective antigen. Proc Natl Acad Sci USA 93:8437–42

Blaustein RO, Koehler TM, Collier RJ, Finkelstein A (1989) Anthrax toxin: channel-forming activity of protective antigen in planar phospholipid bilayers. Proc Natl Acad Sci USA 86:2209–13

Bragg TS, Robertson DL (1989) Nucleotide sequence and analysis of the lethal factor gene (lef) from *Bacillus anthracis*. Gene 81:45–54

Bresnahan PA, Leduc R, Thomas L, Thorner J, Gibson HL, Brake AJ, Barr PJ, Thomas G (1990) Human fur gene encodes a yeast KEX2-like endoprotease that cleaves pro-beta-NGF in vivo. J Cell Biol 111:2851–9

Brossier F, Sirard JC, Guidi-Rontani C, Duflot E, Mock M (1999) Functional analysis of the carboxy-terminal domain of *Bacillus anthracis* protective antigen. Infect Immun 67:964–7

Duesbery NS, Webb CP, Leppla SH, Gordon VM, Klimpel KR, Copeland TD, Ahn NG, Oskarsson MK, Fukasawa K, Paull KD, Vande Woude GF (1998) Proteolytic inactivation of MAP-kinase-kinase by anthrax lethal factor. Science 280: 734–7

Eidels L, Proia RL, Hart DA (1983) Membrane receptors for bacterial toxins. Microbiol Rev 47:596–620

Elliott JL, Mogridge J, Collier RJ (2000) A quantitative study of the interactions of *Bacillus anthracis* edema factor and lethal factor with activated protective antigen. Biochemistry 39:6706–6713

Escuyer V, Collier RJ (1991) Anthrax protective antigen interacts with a specific receptor on the surface of CHO-K1 cells. Infect Immun 59:3381–6

Escuyer V, Duflot E, Sezer O, Danchin A, Mock M (1988) Structural homology between virulence-associated bacterial adenylate cyclases. Gene 71:293–8

Friedlander AM (1986) Macrophages are sensitive to anthrax lethal toxin through an acid-dependent process. J Biol Chem 261:7123–7126

Friedman TC, Gordon VM, Leppla SH, Klimpel KR, Birch NP, Loh YP (1995) In vitro processing of anthrax toxin protective antigen by recombinant PC1 (SPC3) and bovine intermediate lobe secretory vesicle membranes. Arch Biochem Biophys 316:5–13

Gill DM (1978). Seven toxic peptides that cross cell membranes. In Bacterial Toxins and Cell Membranes, J. Jeljaszewicz and T. Wadstrom, eds. (New York: Academic Press), pp 291–332.

Gladstone GP (1946) Immunity to anthrax: protective antigen present in cell-free culture filtrates. Br J Exp Pathol 27:349–418

Goletz TJ, Klimpel KR, Leppla SH, Keith JM, Berzofsky JA (1997) Delivery of antigens to the MHC class I pathway using bacterial toxins. Hum Immunol 54: 129–36

Gordon VM, Klimpel KR, Arora N, Henderson MA, Leppla SH (1995) Proteolytic activation of bacterial toxins by eukaryotic cells is performed by furin and by additional cellular proteases. Infect Immun 63:82–7

Gordon VM, Leppla SH, Hewlett EL (1988) Inhibitors of receptor-mediated endocytosis block the entry of *Bacillus anthracis* adenylate cyclase toxin but not that of *Bordetella pertussis* adenylate cyclase toxin. Infect Immun 56:1066–9

Gordon VM, Rehemtulla A, Leppla SH (1997) A role for PACE4 in the proteolytic activation of anthrax toxin protective antigen. Infect Immun 65:3370–5

Goyard S, Orlando C, Sabatier JM, Labruyere E, d'Alayer J, Fontan G, van Rietschoten J, Mock M, Danchin A, Ullmann A, et al. (1989) Identification of a common domain in calmodulin-activated eukaryotic and bacterial adenylate cyclases. Biochemistry 28:1964–7

Guidi-Rontani C, Weber-Levy M, Mock M, Cabiaux V (2000) Translocation of *Bacillus anthracis* lethal and oedema factors across endosome membranes. Cell Microbiol 2:259–264

Hanna PC, Kruskal BA, Ezekowitz RA, Bloom BR, Collier RJ (1994) Role of macrophage oxidative burst in the action of anthrax lethal toxin. Mol Med 1: 7–18

Klimpel KR, Arora N, Leppla SH (1994) Anthrax toxin lethal factor contains a zinc metalloprotease consensus sequence which is required for lethal toxin activity. Mol Microbiol 13:1093–100

Klimpel KR, Molloy SS, Thomas G, Leppla SH (1992) Anthrax toxin protective antigen is activated by a cell surface protease with the sequence specificity and catalytic properties of furin. Proc Natl Acad Sci USA 89:10277–81

Kochi SK, Martin I, Schiavo G, Mock M, Cabiaux V (1994) The effects of pH on the interaction of anthrax toxin lethal and edema factors with phospholipid vesicles. Biochemistry 33:2604–9

Koehler TM, Collier RJ (1991) Anthrax toxin protective antigen: low-pH-induced hydrophobicity and channel formation in liposomes. Mol Microbiol 5: 1501–6

Labruyere E, Mock M, Ladant D, Michelson S, Gilles AM, Laoide B, Barzu O (1990) Characterization of ATP and calmodulin-binding properties of a truncated form of *Bacillus anthracis* adenylate cyclase. Biochemistry 29:4922–8

Labruyere E, Mock M, Surewicz WK, Mantsch HH, Rose T, Munier H, Sarfati RS, Barzu O (1991) Structural and ligand-binding properties of a truncated form of *Bacillus anthracis* adenylate cyclase and of a catalytically inactive variant in which glutamine substitutes for lysine-346. Biochemistry 30:2619–24

Lacy DB, Tepp W, Cohen AC, DasGupta BR, Stevens RC (1998) Crystal structure of botulinum neurotoxin type A and implications for toxicity. Nat Struct Biol 5: 898–902

Leppla SH (1982a) Anthrax toxin edema factor: a bacterial adenylate cyclase that increase cAMP concentrations in eukaryotic cells. Proc Natl Acad Sci USA 79:3162–3166

Leppla SH (1982b) Anthrax toxin edema factor: a bacterial adenylate cyclase that increases cyclic AMP concentrations of eukaryotic cells. Proc Natl Acad Sci USA 79:3162–6

Leppla SH, Friedlander AM, Cora E (1987). Proteolytic activation of anthrax toxin bound to cellular receptors. In: Bacterial toxins, F. Fehrenbach, J. E. Alouf, P. Falmagne, W. Goebel, J. Jeljaszewicz, D. Jurgens and R. Rappuoli, eds. (Stuttgart, Germany: Gustav Fischer Verlag), pp 111–12.

Little SF, Leppla SH, Burnett JW, Friedlander AM (1994) Structure-function analysis of *Bacillus anthracis* edema factor by using monoclonal antibodies. Biochem Biophys Res Commun 199:676–82

Little SF, Leppla SH, Cora E (1988) Production and characterization of monoclonal antibodies to the protective antigen component of *Bacillus anthracis* toxin. Infect Immun 56:1807–13

Little SF, Novak JM, Lowe JR, Leppla SH, Singh Y, Klimpel KR, Lidgerding BC, Friedlander AM (1996) Characterization of lethal factor binding and cell receptor binding domains of protective antigen of *Bacillus anthracis* using monoclonal antibodies. Microbiology 142:707–15

Menard A, Altendorf K, Breves D, Mock M, Montecucco C (1996) The vacuolar ATPase proton pump is required for the cytotoxicity of *Bacillus anthracis* lethal toxin. FEBS Lett 386:161–4

Mikesell P, Ivins BE, Ristroph JD, Dreier TM (1983) Evidence for plasmid-mediated toxin production in *Bacillus anthracis*. Infect Immun 39:371–376

Miller CJ, Elliott JL, Collier RJ (1999) Anthrax protective antigen: prepore-to-pore conversion. Biochemistry 38:10432–41

Milne JC, Collier RJ (1993) pH-dependent permeabilization of the plasma membrane of mammalian cells by anthrax protective antigen. Mol Microbiol 10:647–53

Milne JC, Furlong D, Hanna PC, Wall JS, Collier RJ (1994) Anthrax protective antigen forms oligomers during intoxication of mammalian cells. J Biol Chem 269: 20607–12

Mock M, Labruyere E, Glaser P, Danchin A, Ullmann A (1988) Cloning and expression of the calmodulin-sensitive *Bacillus anthracis* adenylate cyclase in *Escherichia coli*. Gene 64:77–84

Mogridge J, Mourez M, Collier RJ (2001) Involvement of domain 3 in oligomerization by the protective antigen moiety of anthrax toxin. J Bacteriol, 183:2111–2116

Molloy SS, Bresnahan PA, Leppla SH, Klimpel KR, Thomas G (1992) Human furin is a calcium-dependent serine endoprotease that recognizes the sequence Arg-X-X-Arg and efficiently cleaves anthrax toxin protective antigen. J Biol Chem 267:16396–402

Munier H, Blanco FJ, Precheur B, Diesis E, Nieto JL, Craescu CT, Barzu O (1993) Characterization of a synthetic calmodulin-binding peptide derived from *Bacillus anthracis* adenylate cyclase. J Biol Chem 268:1695–701

Munier H, Bouhss A, Krin E, Danchin A, Gilles AM, Glaser P, Barzu O (1992) The role of histidine 63 in the catalytic mechanism of *Bordetella pertussis* adenylate cyclase. J Biol Chem 267:9816–20

Noskov AN, Kravchenko TB, Noskova VP (1996) [Detection of the functionally active domains in the molecule of protective antigen of the anthrax exotoxin]. Mol Gen Mikrobiol Virusol, 16–20

Novak JM, Stein MP, Little SF, Leppla SH, Friedlander AM (1992) Functional characterization of protease-treated *Bacillus anthracis* protective antigen. J Biol Chem 267:17186–93

Orlando C, d'Alayer J, Baillat G, Castets F, Jeannequin O, Mazie JC, Monneron A (1992) A monoclonal antibody directed against the catalytic site of *Bacillus anthracis* adenylyl cyclase identifies a novel mammalian brain catalytic subunit. Biochemistry 31:3215–22

Petosa C, Collier RJ, Klimpel KR, Leppla SH, Liddington RC (1997) Crystal structure of the anthrax toxin protective antigen. Nature 385:833–8

Pezard C, Berche P, Mock M (1991) Contribution of individual toxin components to virulence of *Bacillus anthracis*. Infect Immun 59:3472–7

Quinn CP, Singh Y, Klimpel KR, Leppla SH (1991) Functional mapping of anthrax toxin lethal factor by in-frame insertion mutagenesis. J Biol Chem 266:20124–30

Robertson DL (1988) Relationships between the calmodulin-dependent adenylate cyclases produced by *Bacillus anthracis* and *Bordetella pertussis*. Biochem Biophys Res Commun 157:1027–32

Robertson DL, Leppla SH (1986) Molecular cloning and expression in *Escherichia coli* of the lethal factor gene of *Bacillus anthracis*. Gene 44:71–78

Robertson DL, Tippetts MT, Leppla SH (1988) Nucleotide sequence of the *Bacillus anthracis* edema factor gene (cya): a calmodulin-dependent adenylate cyclase. Gene 73:363–71

Sellman BR, Nassi S, Collier RJ (2001) Point mutations in anthrax protective antigen that block translocation. J Biol Chem, 276:8371–8376

Singh Y, Chaudhary VK, Leppla SH (1989) A deleted variant of *Bacillus anthracis* protective antigen is non-toxic and blocks anthrax toxin action in vivo. J Biol Chem 264:19103–7

Singh Y, Klimpel KR, Arora N, Sharma M, Leppla SH (1994) The chymotrypsin-sensitive site, FFD315, in anthrax toxin protective antigen is required for translocation of lethal factor. J Biol Chem 269:29039–46

Singh Y, Klimpel KR, Quinn CP, Chaudhary VK, Leppla SH (1991) The carboxyl-terminal end of protective antigen is required for receptor binding and anthrax toxin activity. J Biol Chem 266:15493–7

Smith H, Keppie J, Stanley JL (1955) The chemical basis of the virulence of *Bacillus anthracis*. V. The specific toxin produced by *B. anthracis* in vivo. Br J Exp Pathol 36:460–472

Song L, Hobaugh MR, Shustak C, Cheley S, Bayley H, Gouaux JE (1996) Structure of staphylococcal alpha-hemolysin, a heptameric transmembrane pore. Science 274:1859–66

Stanley JL, Smith H (1961) Purification of factor I and recognition of a third factor of the anthrax toxin. J Gen Microbiol 26:49–66

Tang G, Leppla SH (1999) Proteasome activity is required for anthrax lethal toxin to kill macrophages. Infect Immun 67:3055–60

Tippetts MT, Robertson DL (1988) Molecular cloning and expression of the *Bacillus anthracis* edema factor toxin gene: a calmodulin-dependent adenylate cyclase. J Bacteriol 170:2263–6

Varughese M, Teixeira AV, Liu S, Leppla SH (1999) Identification of a receptor-binding region within domain 4 of the protective antigen component of anthrax toxin. Infect Immun 67:1860–5

Vitale G, Pellizzari R, Recchi C, Napolitani G, Mock M, Montecucco C (1998) Anthrax lethal factor cleaves the N-terminus of MAPKKs and induces tyrosine/threonine phosphorylation of MAPKs in cultured macrophages. Biochem Biophys Res Commun 248:706–11

Vodkin MH, Leppla SH (1983) Cloning of the protective antigen gene of *Bacillus anthracis*. Cell 34:693–7

Wang XM, Mock M, Ruysschaert JM, Cabiaux V (1996) Secondary structure of anthrax lethal toxin proteins and their interaction with large unilamellar vesicles: a fourier-transform infrared spectroscopy approach. Biochemistry 35: 14939–46

Wang XM, Wattiez R, Brossier F, Mock M, Falmagne P, Ruysschaert JM, Cabiaux V (1998) Use of a photoactivatable lipid to probe the topology of PA63 of *Bacillus anthracis* in lipid membranes. Eur J Biochem 256:179–83

Wang XM, Wattiez R, Mock M, Falmagne P, Ruysschaert JM, Cabiaux V (1997) Structure and interaction of PA63 and EF (edema toxin) of *Bacillus anthracis* with lipid membrane. Biochemistry 36:14906–13

Welkos SL, Lowe JR, Eden-McCutchan F, Vodkin M, Leppla SH, Schmidt JJ (1988) Sequence and analysis of the DNA encoding protective antigen of *Bacillus anthracis*. Gene 69:287–300

Wesche J, Elliott JL, Falnes PO, Olsnes S, Collier RJ (1998) Characterization of membrane translocation by anthrax protective antigen. Biochemistry 37: 15737–46

Xia ZG, Storm DR (1990) A-type ATP binding consensus sequences are critical for the catalytic activity of the calmodulin-sensitive adenylyl cyclase from *Bacillus anthracis*. J Biol Chem 265:6517–20

Note Added in Proof. Since the original submission of this manuscript in July of 2000, many exciting advances in the field of anthrax toxin research have occurred. We refer interested readers to the following articles:

Bradley KA, Mogridge J, Mourez M, Collier RJ, Young, JA (2001) Identification of the cellular receptor for anthrax toxin. Nature 414:225–229

Drum CL, Yan SZ, Bard J, Shen YQ, Lu D, Soelaiman S, Grabarek Z, Bohm A, Tang WJ (2002) Structural basis for the activation of anthrax adenylyl cyclase exotoxin by calmodulin. Nature 415:396–402

MOUREZ M, KANE RS, MOGRIDGE J, METALLO S, DESCHATELETS P, SELLMAN BR, WHITESIDES GM, COLLIER RJ (2001) Designing a polyvalent inhibitor of anthrax toxin. Nat Biotechnol 19:958–961

PANNIFER AD, WONG TY, SCHWARZENBACHER R, RENATUS M, PETOSA C, BIENKOWSKA J, LACY DB, COLLIER RJ, PARK S, LEPPLA SH, HANNA P, LIDDINGTON RC (2001) Crystal structure of the anthrax lethal factor. Nature 414:229–233

SELLMAN BR, MOUREZ M, COLLIER RJ (2001) Dominant-negative mutants of a toxin subunit: an approach to therapy of anthrax. Science 292:695–697

CHAPTER 5

Bacillus anthracis Cell Envelope Components

A. FOUET, S. MESNAGE

Abstract. *Bacillus anthracis* is a Gram-positive bacterium harboring a complex parietal architecture. The cytoplasmic membrane is surrounded by a thick peptidoglycan of the A1γ type. Only one associated polymer, a polysaccharide composed of galactose, *N*-acetylglucosamine, and *N*-acetylmannosamine, is covalently linked to the peptidoglycan. Outside the cell wall is an S-layer. Two proteins can each compose the S-layer. They are noncovalently anchored to the cell wall polysaccharide by their SLH N-ter-

A. FOUET, S. MESNAGE
Toxines et Pathogénie Bactériennes (URA 2172, CNRS), Institut Pasteur, 28 rue du Dr Roux, 75724, Paris cédex 15, France.
Present address: S. MESNAGE, Laboratoire de Recherche Moléculaire sur les Antibiotiques (L.R.M.A.), 15 rue de l'Ecole de Médecine, 75270 Paris cédex 05, France. Email: afouet@pasteur.fr.

minal domain. The poly-γ-D-glutamate capsule, which covers the S-layer, has an antiphagocytic role and its synthesis is dependent on environmental factors mimicking the mammalian host, such as bicarbonate and a temperature of 37 °C.

1 Introduction

Bacillus anthracis is a Gram-positive sporulating bacterium. It is therefore found either as vegetative cells or as spores. The Gram-positive classification depends on a long-established cytological reaction (the Gram stain), which differentiates surface structures into two major types (Salton 1964). The multilayered structure of the cell wall allows Gram-positive bacteria to retain a crystal precipitate in the presence of solvents whereas Gram-negative bacteria do not. Gram-negative bacteria, unlike Gram-positive bacteria, have an outer membrane outside the peptidoglycan.

This chapter describes the *B. anthracis* surface envelope components, from the inside to the outside of the bacterium. Unfortunately, some of the cell wall components in *B. anthracis* have not been studied. Therefore, when appropriate, data from closely related organisms, i.e., other *Bacillus* species, will be summarized to give an idea of what the *B. anthracis* surface might be. The surface of *B. anthracis* is unique. In addition to the classic cytoplasmic membrane and peptidoglycan layers, *B. anthracis* has two structures which are not present on the surface of all bacteria, namely an S-layer and a capsule. Indeed, very few bacteria possess both of these structures. The complexity of the parietal architecture of *B. anthracis* and the possible structural or functional complementarity of these structures makes this topic particularly interesting.

2 Cytoplasmic Membrane

The cytoplasmic membrane is the least studied of all *B. anthracis* envelope components. Even that of *B. subtilis* has not been extensively analyzed, despite the advantage that the presence of a single membrane gives to experimentalists (de Mendoza et al. 1993 and references therein).

The membrane is composed of phospholipids and fatty acids. Eighty percent of *B. subtilis* phospholipids are of the common bacterial lipids, mostly phosphatidylglycerol, and some phosphatidylethanolamine

(Bishop et al. 1967; Guffanti et al. 1987). Direct data and supposition suggest that the phospholipids and glycolipid synthetic pathways are probably similar to those documented in other organisms (Lennarz 1970). Acyl-acyl carrier proteins transfer acyl groups in successive steps. However, the regulation of lipid biosynthetic enzymes by an "on or off" transcriptional regulatory system rather than modulation of enzyme activity might be specific to *Bacillus*. The implication of an "extra cytoplasmic factor" (ECF) transcriptional factor such as σ^X in the synthesis of lipid synthetic enzymes will also have to be analyzed. For instance, in *B. subtilis*, the expression of σ^X modifies the ratio between negatively charged and neutral phospholipids and consequently the sensitivity of the bacterium to positively charged antibiotics (Huang and Helmann 1998).

Iso- and anteiso-branched fatty acids are the major components of the lipids in *Bacillus* species (Kaneda 1991). Branched-chain fatty acids are generally, but not always, more abundant than straight-chain acids. In *B. anthracis* whole cells, hexadecanoic acid and tetradecanoic acid are the most abundant when strains are grown on complex medium, and branched-chain fatty acids make up less than a third of the total. Interestingly, the content of branched fatty acids rises to over two-thirds when strains are grown on synthetic media (Lawrence et al. 1991). The fatty acid biosynthesis activities depend on acyl carrier proteins (Vanden Boom and Cronan Jr. 1989). The synthesis pathway may be diversified. The ratio between branched- and straight-chain fatty acids could be due to the relative affinities of the condensing enzymes for acetyl-CoA or acyl-CoA esters, respectively (de Mendoza et al. 1993). Also, the fatty acid composition of the bacterial phospholipids is modified in response to growth temperature, with more low-melting-point fatty acids being incorporated into membrane lipids when the temperature decreases (de Mendoza and Farias 1988). Major changes in membrane structure occur during spore formation. It is therefore plausible that the fatty acid composition also changes during this differentiation step.

Knowledge about the lipid biosynthetic pathways and their regulation is now accumulating in *B. subtilis*. Genomic comparisons and searches for homologs in *B. anthracis* will rapidly identify gross similarities or differences between *B. anthracis* and other species.

Membrane-associated polysaccharides (lipoteichoic acids) are found in *B. subtilis* and in some *Bacillus cereus* strains (Iwasaki et al. 1989). However, we have found no report of lipoteichoic acids in *B. anthracis*, and their absence from other *Bacillus* has been reported. It is therefore plausible that *B. anthracis* does not synthesize such polymers.

Lipoproteins are membrane-associated components. They are covalently linked to the cytoplasmic membrane, a cysteine residue being bound to fatty acids. The cysteine residue is part of a consensus sequence (L a g C). Sixteen proteins harboring this motif have been found in *B. subtilis.* The presence of lipoproteins has also been described in *B. cereus.* The association with the membrane concentrates their enzymatic activities at the surface of the bacterium. The variety of the activities of membrane-associated enzymes in other species (iron captation, peptide transport, initiation of sporulation, cytochrome oxidase activity, osmoprotectant transport, β-lactamase) indicates that identifying such proteins in *B. anthracis* would be of great interest. Fifteen ORFs have been identified in the genomic sequence as containing the consensus sequence in their N-terminal region (T. Read, personal communication) and are obvious candidates for such studies.

3 Peptidoglycan

The peptidoglycan layer is typically much thicker in Gram-positive bacteria than in Gram-negative species. In Gram-positive bacteria, it can be visualized by electron microscopy and appears as an amorphous structure, 20–50 nm thick and apposed to the underlying cytoplasmic membrane. It protects the underlying protoplast, resists turgor, and maintains the shape of the cell. Because of the absence of an outer membrane, the peptidoglycan layer may block unrestricted movement of materials between the cytoplasmic membrane and the environment. The cell wall is involved in cation binding, in maintaining an optimum ionic environment for membrane-bound enzyme systems, and in immobilizing specific proteins.

3.1 Composition and Structure

The cell wall is composed of peptidoglycan *stricto sensu* and of associated polymers. The peptidoglycan is a complex heteropolysaccharide made of glycan chains that are linked by small peptides. It is a single molecule that completely covers the bacterium like a net, and it can constitute up to 40% of the cell wall mass.

The glycan chain consists of alternating units of *N*-acetylglucosamine and *N*-acetylmuramic acid held together by *β*1->4 glycosidic linkages (Fig. 1A) (GHUYSEN 1968). The glycan chains are connected to short "stem" peptides through amide linkages between the carboxyl groups on muramyl residues and the terminal amino groups of the peptides. The stem peptides are linked through alternating L- and D-amino acid centers. In most *Bacillus* species, the stem peptide contains an N-terminal L-Ala with its carboxyl group linked to the amino group of D-Glu. The *γ* carboxyl group of this D-Glu is linked to the amino group at the L-center of meso-

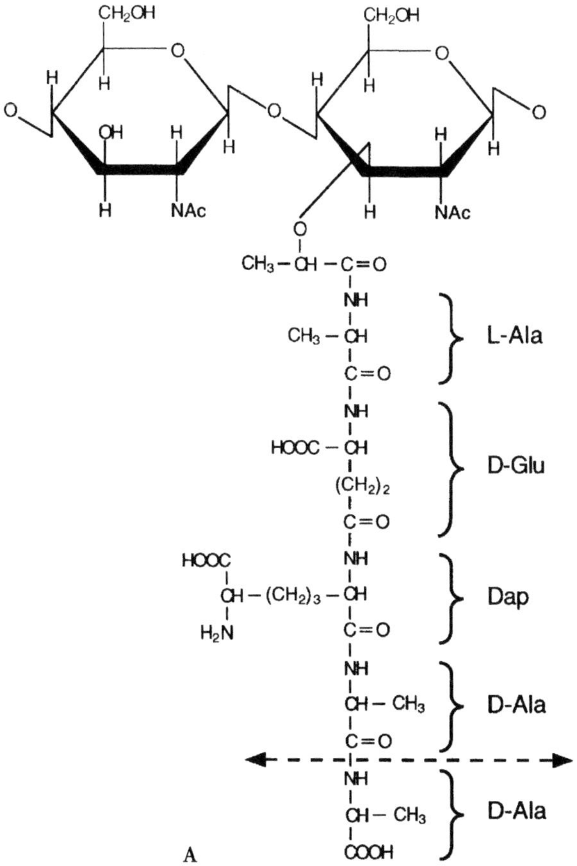

A

Fig. 1. Schematic representation of a type *A1γ* peptidoglycan precursor (**A**) and of the specificity of peptidoglycan hydrolytic enzymes (**B**, see next page)

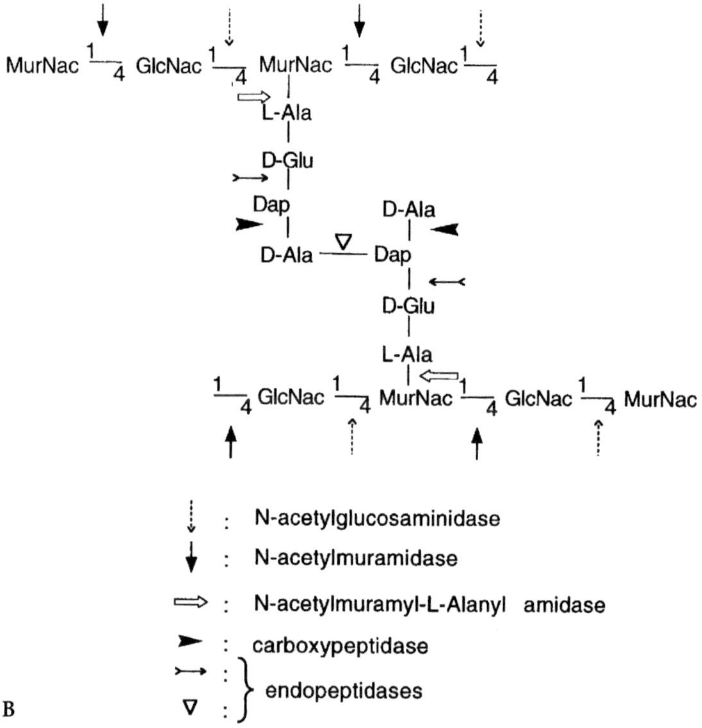

Fig. 1B

DAP, and the carboxyl group at this center is linked to D-Ala D-Ala. The type of cross-linkage and the identity of the amino acid at position 3 have been used as chemotaxonomic markers (Schleifer and Kandler 1972). That of *B. anthracis* is of the A1γ type. A designates a cross-linkage between positions 3 and 4 of the peptide units, 1 that it is a direct cross-linkage, and γ that the linkage is to DAP (Fig. 1A).

The peptidoglycan is thus made up of stacks of glycan chains, one above the other (Graham and Beveridge 1994).

3.2 Synthesis and Turnover

Precursors are inserted into the peptidoglycan outside of the cytoplasmic membrane (Pooley 1976). Peptidoglycan biosynthesis takes place in three stages in three different subcellular compartments: the cytosol, the interface between the cytosol and the membrane, and outside the membrane.

In the cytosol, the reaction of phosphoenolpyruvate and UDP-*N*-acetyl glucosamine gives rise to UDP-*N*-acetyl muramic acid. The five amino acid residues are then sequentially linked to the lactyl group of the UDP-*N*-acetyl muramic acid in four steps; first, L-Ala, then D-Glu and DAP, and finally the dipeptide D-Ala D-Ala.

At the interface between the cytosol and the membrane, the UDP-*N*-acetyl muramic pentapeptide is covalently linked to a lipid transporter. *N*-acetyl glucosamine is added from UDP-*N*-acetyl glucosamine to this molecule, termed lipid I, giving rise to lipid II.

Lipid II is then transferred to the outside of the membrane, and the precursor is integrated into the glycan chain. However, it cannot be excluded that the elongation of the glycan chain occurs before the translocation step (SHOCKMAN and BARRETT 1983).

The monomers are linked to the preexisting polymer by high-molecular-weight penicillin-binding proteins. Simultaneous with its incorporation into the peptidoglycan, the precursor pentapeptide is converted into a tetrapeptide by elimination of the terminal D-Ala residue. However, the proportion of di-, tri-, and tetrapeptides varies, depending on the wall cross-linking. The peptide is cross-linked if the transpeptidation acceptor is DAP or it is not if it is water: in *B. anthracis*, only 19% is cross-linked (ZIPPERLE JR. et al. 1984).

The *Bacillus* peptidoglycan is thick, and its diameter is constant during vegetative growth. This suggests that there is a synchronization between biosynthesis on the cytoplasmic side and degradation on the outside of the cell. This coordination has to be temporal and spatial.

Several peptidoglycan hydrolases (glycosidases or peptidases) have been described, among which only those hydrolytic enzymes detrimental to peptidoglycan integrity are called autolysins. Depending on the enzymatic activity, N- or C-amino terminal groups (amidases, endopeptidases) or reducing groups (muramidases, glucosaminidases) are released after peptidoglycan cleavage (Fig. 1 B). Few hydrolytic enzymes have been characterized in bacteria of the *Bacillus* genus (SMITH et al. 1996; for review, see SHOCKMAN and HÖLTJE 1994). The analysis of the complete genomic sequence of *B. subtilis* suggests the existence of many hydrolases possibly involved in peptidoglycan synthesis: 12 amidases, 4 carboxypeptidases, 1 glucosaminidase, 3 hydrolytic enzymes of unknown specificity, and 13 penicillin-binding proteins (KUNST et al. 1997). The complexity of the rp-HPLC pattern obtained after peptidoglycan digestion suggests that there are many endogenous enzymatic activities (ATRIH et al. 1998).

Similar biochemical, genetic, and genomic analyses have yet to be carried out on *B. anthracis* peptidoglycan.

In *B. subtilis*, peptidoglycan hydrolysis is controlled both at the genetic and the enzymatic levels. Two sigma transcription factors (σ^A and σ^D) are involved in the expression of different autolysins (Haldenwang 1995). Various hydrolases act at different phases of development, and the expression of their genes is under the control of transcriptional factors that are dependent on phase development (Kuroda et al. 1993; Sekiguchi et al. 1995).

Electrochemical and pH gradients are important for the inactivation of the autolysins (Jolliffe et al. 1981). Thus these enzymes are active on the outer peptidoglycan layers but inactive in the vicinity of the naturally energized cytoplasmic membrane. This is in agreement with the model suggesting that peptidoglycan growth is from the inside to the outside (Koch and Doyle 1985; Merad et al. 1989; Hancock 1997). In fact, three zones can be distinguished: an internal portion where monomers are incorporated, a middle zone, and an outside zone that undergoes a hydrolysis (Koch and Doyle 1985; Doyle and Koch 1987). This way, the peptidoglycan is degraded where necessary for cell growth but is kept intact where its protective function is required. Some of the biochemical properties of the cell wall inhibit hydrolytic activities. For instance, the amino groups of the amino sugars can be substituted or not, and in *B. anthracis*, only 12% of the glucosamine and 66% of the muramic acid are *N*-acetylated. This low acetylation accounts for resistance of the *B. anthracis* cell wall to lysozyme (Zipperle Jr. et al. 1984).

3.3 Associated Polymers

Gram-positive bacteria synthesize anionic polymers that are covalently linked to the peptidoglycan. They are grouped in three categories according to their biochemical composition: (a) teichoic acids, which are polyolphosphates, (b) teichuronic acids, which are uronic acids containing polysaccharides, and (c) acidic or neutral polysaccharides, which cannot be classified as belonging to one of the other two groups. In *B. subtilis*, there is a genetic control such that depending on the phosphate concentration, teichoic acids or teichuronic acids are synthesized (Ellwood and Tempest 1972; Hancock 1983; Soldo et al. 1999). The extremely low phosphate content of the *B. anthracis* cell wall makes the presence of teichoic acids extremely improbable (Molnár and Prágai 1971). In fact, only a neutral polysaccharide has been found linked to the peptidoglycan. It was initially described in 1922 and has been the object of many studies since (Kramar 1922; Burger 1950). However, its composition became known only recently with the development of new analysis techniques. It has a molecular mass of 12 kDa and is composed of galactose, *N*-acetylglucosamine, and *N*-acetylmannosamine (Ekwunife et al. 1991; Fox et al. 1993). The ratio for these three constituents appears to vary. The initial report mentioned 3:2:1. However, we have found a slightly different ratio of 10:3:1 (Mesnage et al. 2000). This polysaccharide is immunogenic and permits the indirect identification of *B. anthracis*, through the Ascoli test, described at the beginning of the twentieth century (Ascoli 1911). This test is still used, and it indicates the presence, in body fluids or tissues, of antibodies directed against *B. anthracis*. Monoclonal antibodies to this polysaccharide were developed and characterized during the search for tools for differentiation of *B. anthracis* from closely related *Bacillus thuringiensis* and *B. cereus* species (Ezzell Jr. et al. 1990). The interaction of these monoclonal antibodies with the galactose-*N*-acetylglucosamine polysaccharide is inhibited by galactose. The functions of *B. anthracis* cell wall-associated polysaccharide are discussed in Sect. 4.2.

4
S-layer

When *B. anthracis* does not produce a capsule, its cell wall appears layered (Fig. 2; Gerhardt 1967; Holt and Leadbetter 1969). The layer surrounding the peptidoglycan is composed of fragments displaying a highly patterned ultrastructure and has been termed the S-layer, for surface layer. S-layers are proteinaceous paracrystalline sheaths, which completely cover the cell surface. They are found ubiquitously, being present on the surface of many archaea and bacteria (for review, see Sleytr and Messner 1983; Sleytr et al. 1993, 1996). Most result from noncovalent entropy-driven assembly of a single (glyco)protein protomer on the surface of the bacteria. Various functions have been proposed for S-layers, and they may be a virulence factor (Kotiranta et al. 1998; Messner and Sleytr 1992).

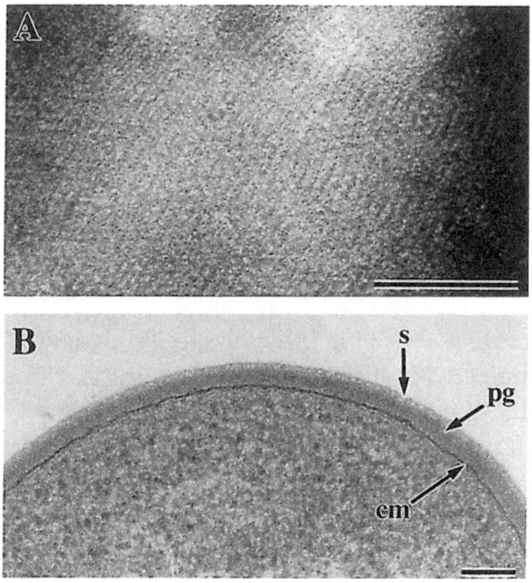

Fig. 2A,B. *Bacillus anthracis* S-layer. Negative staining of *B. anthracis* S-layer fragments from a plasmid-free strain (**A**) and of a thin section from the same strain (**B**). *s*, S-layer; *pg*, peptidoglycan; *cm*, cytoplasmic membrane. Bar, 100 nm

4.1
Composition, Genetics

It was first suggested that a major bacterial protein often very abundant in *B. anthracis* culture supernatants was an S-layer component. This 94-kDa protein is produced by various virulent and plasmid-free strains of *B. anthracis* and must therefore be chromosomally encoded. The N-terminal sequence of this protein, Sap (surface array protein), and those of polypeptides obtained by limited chymotrypsin digestion, were determined. Oligonucleotide probes were thus designed and used to isolate *sap*. This gene was disrupted, and no other 94-kDa protein was observed in the culture supernatant of this mutant (Etienne-Toumelin et al. 1995). However, the *Δsap* mutant still possessed an S-layer and an abundant 94-kDa protein, EA1 (extractable antigen 1) (Ezzell Jr. and Abshire 1988), in its pellet fraction (Mesnage et al. 1997). By an approach similar to that used for *sap*, the *eag* gene, encoding EA1, was isolated. The genes *sap* and *eag* map close together on the chromosome and were deleted together or independently (Fig. 3A). Sap and EA1 are both S-layer constituents, and

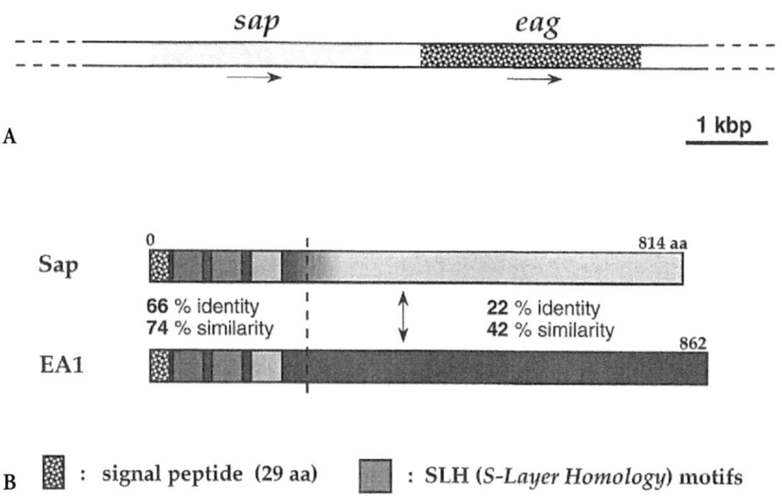

Fig. 3. **A** Genetic organization of the two *B. anthracis* S-layer genes. **B** Schematic comparison of the two *B. anthracis* S-layer proteins

there is no other S-layer component, because structured layers were visible on all the strains except the double deleted mutant. *sap* and *eag* are in the same orientation, separated by a noncoding fragment of approximately 700 bp, *eag* following *sap*. They are organized as independent transcriptional units (Mignot et al. 2002).

The deduced amino acid sequences of Sap (814 residues) and EA1 (862 residues) show common features (Fig. 3B). Both proteins harbor a classic Gram-positive signal peptide (Simonen and Palva 1993). In each case, the mature protein starts with three SLH (S-layer homology) motifs of 50 residues each. In fact, these two proteins are very similar along the 200 first residues. After this region, the proteins differ appreciably. When subjected to proteinase K proteolysis, these proteins each yielded a protease resistant core, corresponding to the C-terminal domain and starting at residue 211 for both proteins (Mesnage et al. 1999a). Thus these proteins could be composed of two domains: the first, constituted by the SLH motifs, is discussed in Sect. 4.2; the second, the protease resistant core, may be the crystallization domain. This hypothesis is currently under investigation.

The existence of two S-layer genes may result in the simultaneous synthesis of both proteins or in the activation of the second gene if one is deleted. For example, in some Gram-positive bacteria, including *Bacillus stearothermophilus*, more than one S-layer can appear sequentially (Sára et al. 1996). In other cases, e.g., *Clostridium perfringens*, *Clostridium difficile*, and *Bacillus brevis*, two proteins are synthesized simultaneously in abundance (Tsuboi et al. 1982; Kawata et al. 1984; Takumi et al. 1991). In *B. anthracis*, both proteins are present on the surface of the bacteria. EA1 is nearly exclusively cell associated, whereas Sap is equally cell associated and released into the supernatant. The presence of both a signal peptide and SLH motifs in these proteins is consistent with the cell surface localization.

To determine whether both S-layer components are produced in vivo, the presence of anti-EA1 and anti-Sap antibodies was tested in sera from mice infected with *B. anthracis* spores. Antibodies to both were detected, indicating that the surface proteins EA1 and Sap are both major surface antigens and are synthesized in vivo (Mesnage et al. 1997, 1998). That which is exclusively cell associated yielded the most intense signal and is therefore EA1, the major extractable antigen described by Ezzell and Abshire (Ezzell Jr. and Abshire 1988).

4.2 Anchoring

There are at least 18 ORFs with SLH sequences in *B. anthracis*; at least 15 on the chromosome, 2 on pXO1, and 1 on pXO2 (www.tigr.org, and accession numbers AF065404 and AF188935, respectively). SLH motifs have been found in many surface proteins from Gram-positive bacteria and have been suggested to be responsible for cell wall binding (Lupas et al. 1994; Lemaire et al. 1995; Ries et al. 1997; Sára et al. 1996; Olabarría et al. 1996). This has been confirmed by studies with *B. anthracis* S-layer proteins (Chauvaux et al. 1999; Mesnage et al. 1999a,b). The three motifs of EA1 and Sap can be produced in large amounts as stable His-tagged polypeptides in *E. coli*, consistent with the idea that they form a structural domain (Chauvaux et al. 1999; Mesnage et al. 1999a). These polypeptides are able to bind *B. anthracis* purified cell wall in vitro, with the same high affinity (K_D 10^{-7} M). It is likely that they are responsible for the cell wall targeting of the S-layer proteins (Chauvaux et al. 1999; Mesnage et al. 1999a). The SLH domains are unable to bind hydrofluoric acid-treated cell walls (Mesnage et al. 1999 a), indicating that they bind to a secondary polymer, possibly the neutral polysaccharide, covalently linked to the peptidoglycan, described by Ekwunife et al. (Ekwunife et al. 1991). The S-layer extraction properties indicate that the binding of the SLH domain to the polysaccharide is non-covalent. Chimeric genes encoding fusion proteins combining the SLH domains of EA1 or Sap and the mature form of normally secreted proteins (the *B. subtilis* levansucrase, or a fragment of the *Clostridium tetanii* toxin) have been constructed and inserted into *B. anthracis* chromosome. The recombinant strains display the chimeric proteins at their surface. Furthermore, the first strain displays saccharolytic activity on its surface. Protection against challenge with lethal doses of tetanus toxin is observed when the second strain is used to vaccinate mice. Thus the SLH domains are sufficient to anchor proteins in their active form and consequently the S-layer proteins, to the surface of the bacilli (Mesnage et al. 2000).

A bicistronic operon (*csaAB*) involved in the biosynthesis of the peptidoglycan-associated polysaccharide has been identified. A mutant in the distal gene is unable to anchor S-layer proteins and also many other SLH-containing proteins. The parental and mutant strain peptidoglycans are similar. The peptidoglycan-associated polysaccharides of the parental and mutant strains have the same molecular mass, and the same composition, as analyzed by gas chromatography. However, ion-exchange chromatography purification of polysaccharide extracts revealed that a parental negatively charged fraction is absent from the Δ*csaB* mutant. Enzymatic assays and RMN analysis indicate that this modification corresponds to the addition of pyruvate residues. Contrary to its pyruvylated counterpart, the nonpyruvylated polysaccharide is unable to bind SLH domains. CsaB is responsible for the pyruvylation of the polysaccharide and consequently for the anchoring of the numerous SLH-containing proteins of *B. anthracis*. The *csaB* mutant bacilli have a twisted filamentous morphology. This is the consequence of a great reduction in autolysis activity, probably due to SLH-containing autolysins not being anchored in the appropriate site (Mesnage et al. 2000).

5 Capsule

The first description of *B. anthracis* capsule goes back to M'Fadyean's work in 1903. This author described a method for coloring the germs present in animals presumed to have died from anthrax. An aqueous solution of methylene blue yields a "violet-stained substance" found mainly in proximity of the bacilli. This technique is still used to identify *B. anthracis* in the field (Lindeque and Turnbull 1994; Quinn and Turnbull 1998). The capsule can also be visualized by electron microscopy (Fig. 4).

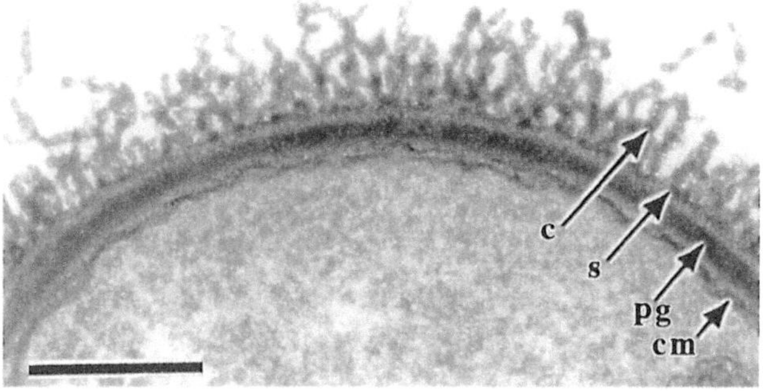

Fig. 4. Envelope component visualization on a capsulated *B. anthracis* strain by negative staining of a thin section. *s*, S-layer; *pg*, peptidoglycan; *cm*, cytoplasmic membrane; *c*, capsule. Bar, 250 nm

M'Fadyean also noted that the violet reaction was not obtained with artificial cultures of the bacilli. In the following years, Preisz described the relationship between in vivo formation of the capsule and *B. anthracis* virulence (Preisz 1909). He showed that capsulated strains are virulent, whereas noncapsulated strains are avirulent. A few years later, Bail suggested that the capsule may constitute an "agressine" (Bail 1915). *B. anthracis* capsule is currently defined as one of its two major virulence factors (Thorne 1993).

5.1 Composition and Structure

The capsule was purified and shown to be a polypeptide in 1933 (Tomcsik and Szongott 1933). It was identified as being a polymer of D-glutamic acid (Ivánovics and Brückner 1937a, b). In *B. anthracis* the glutamyl polypeptide adheres to the cell, whereas in other organisms a similar polypeptide is released into the medium (Avakyan et al. 1965; Tomcsik 1956). This suggests that, in *B. anthracis*, the anchoring mechanism, its eventual components, will have to be analyzed. Finally, it was established that the linkage between the D-glutamic acid residues constituting the capsule of in vitro-grown *B. anthracis* is of the γ- and not of the α type as initially believed (Fig. 5A) (Hanby and Rydon 1946; Brückner and Kovacs 1953). Thus the glutamic acid residues are mainly bound by peptide bonds between γ-carboxyl and α-amino groups, and this was shown also to be the case in vivo (Zwartouw and Smith 1956). The size of poly-

A

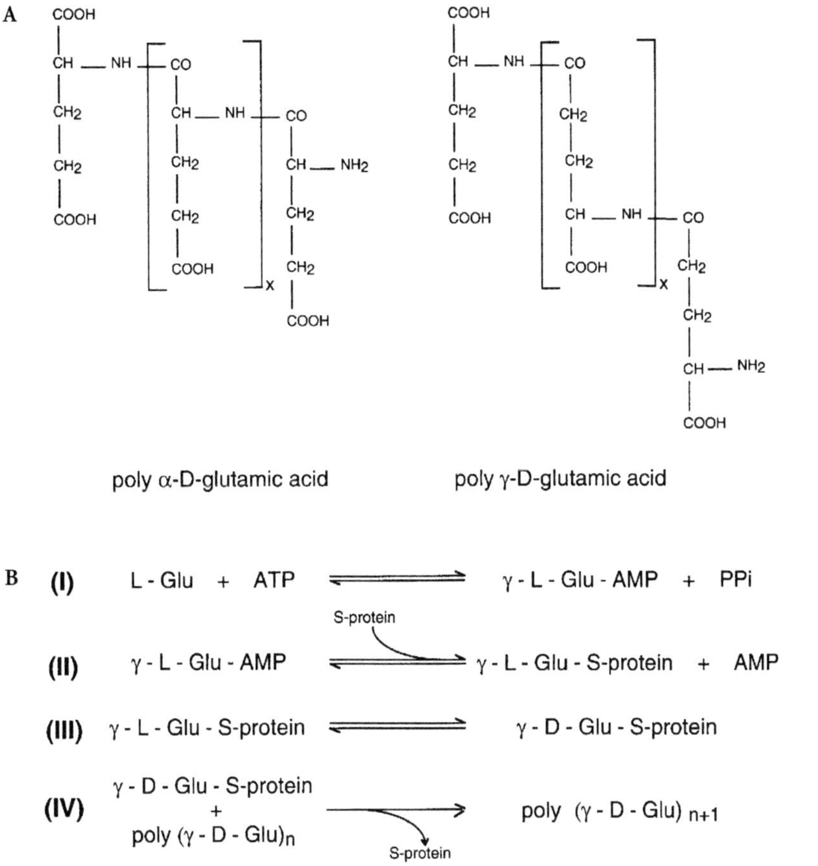

Fig. 5 A, B. Structure and biosynthesis of *B. anthracis* capsule. **A** Compared structure of poly-α-D- and poly-γ-D-glutamic acids. **B** Biosynthetic pathway of *B. licheniformis* capsule as described by TROY (TROY 1973 a, b)

glutamic chains seems to differ depending on the growth conditions of the bacilli: in vitro they are between 20 and 55 kDa (HANBY and RYDON 1946; BRÜCKNER and KOVACS 1953; GOODMAN and NITECKI 1967), whereas in vivo they contain thousands of residues with an estimated molecular mass of 215 kDa (RECORD and WALLIS 1956). The cohesion of the capsule is dependent on both divalent cations (Mg^{2+}, Ca^{2+}), which link the acidic groups of the polymers, and hydration (BEVERIDGE and GRAHAM 1991).

Although peptide capsule is not common, some bacteria, including *B. subtilis*, *Bacillus megaterium*, and *Bacillus licheniformis*, synthesize glutamic acid polymers (Tomcsik 1956; König and Niemetz 1997). It can either be a constituent of the cell wall or be secreted into the medium. These polymers are composed of D- or L-isomers bound by α or γ linkages (for review, see König and Niemetz 1997). Some bacteria, such as *B. licheniformis*, synthesize two polymers, one composed of the D- and one of the L-isomer (Thorne and Leonard 1958). The biochemical structures of *B. anthracis* and *B. licheniformis* capsules are identical, and the same precursor is used for their synthesis, namely, L-glutamic acid (Thorne 1956; Leonard and Housewright 1963). This suggests that their biosynthesis pathways are also identical.

5.2 Biosynthesis

The only species in which polypeptide biosynthesis has been thoroughly studied is *B. licheniformis*. The polyglutamic acid synthetase activity was demonstrated in disrupted cells (Leonard and Housewright 1963). L-Glutamic acid is the precursor of both D- and L-glutamic acids incorporated into the polymer, and D-glutamic acid is not an intermediate. The synthesis of the poly-γ-D-glutamic acid is by a membranous enzymatic complex and can be described in three steps (Fig. 5B; Troy 1973a, b; Gardner and Troy 1979).

During the first step, in the presence of L-glutamic acid, Mg^{2+}, and hydroxylamine, a membranous glutamyl-activating enzyme catalyzes the ATP-dependent formation of glutamyl hydroxamate. In the absence of hydroxylamine, a γ-L-glutamyl adenylate residue is formed (Fig. 5B, I). The D-isomer is not a precursor for this enzymatic reaction. Subsequent to the activation step, the γ-L-glutamyl adenylate is converted into a γ-D-glutamyl adenyl residue. A protein-bound thioester may be a second intermediate in this process (Fig. 5B, II and III). The last step is the transfer of the activated glutamic acid to an endogenous membrane-bound poly(γ-D-glutamyl) acceptor (Fig. 5B, IV). Thus the polyglutamyl chains are extended by sequential addition of new glutamyl residues to the terminal amino group of a glutamyl residue of the acceptor.

A major difference between *B. anthracis* and *B. licheniformis*, with respect to poly-γ-D-glutamic acid synthesis, is the requirement for bicarbonate in *B. anthracis*. However, its role is not that of a carbon source, but of a regulatory factor (Eastin and Thorne 1963; Meynell and Meynell 1964, 1966; see the chapter by T.M. Koehler, this volume).

In *B. anthracis*, capsule synthesis is encoded by the plasmid pXO2 (Green et al. 1985; Uchida et al. 1985). This was proven by elegant genetic experiments using transduction and mating systems (Green et al. 1985). Cells of *B. cereus* and of *B. anthracis* previously cured for pXO2 became Cap^+ after they received pXO2. A DNA region was cloned and shown to be sufficient for poly-γ-D-glutamic acid synthesis but not for the production of wild-type amounts of capsular material in recombinant bacteria (Makino et al. 1989; see the chapter by T.M. Koehler, this volume). This region contains most of a four-gene operon (Makino et al. 1989; Uchida et al. 1993). The first three genes, *capB*, *capC*, and *capA* encode the synthetic enzymes of molecular masses 44.8, 16.5, and 46.4 kDa, respectively. They appear to be membrane-associated enzymes. Interestingly, *B. subtilis* strain 168, the genome of which was sequenced, harbors *cap* gene homologs, namely *ywsC*, *ywtA*, and *ywtB* (Kunst et al. 1997). However, the synthesis of glutamyl-polypeptide immunologically related to that of *B. anthracis* has not been described in that strain. Three genes encoding a poly-γ-glutamate synthetic (PGS) system of another *B. subtilis* strain, which secretes poly-γ-D- and poly-γ-L-glutamic acids, were cloned (Ashiuchi et al. 1999). These genes, *pgsBCA*, are almost identical to the *B. subtilis* 168 genes and are very similar to the *B. anthracis capBCA* genes. Interestingly, coexpression of a glutamate racemase in *E. coli* cells harboring *pgsBCA* increased both the polymer production and the proportion of D-isomer content. This suggests that the PGS system does not include a component for glutamate isomerization. Although it is not necessarily the case, the sequence analogy indicates that the situation might be similar with the proteins encoded by *capBCA*. Unfortunately, no specific enzymatic function has been assigned to any of these *B. anthracis* or *B. subtilis* proteins. The only indication is that PgsB possesses a consensus sequence found in the amide ligase superfamily. The fourth gene of the *B. anthracis cap* operon, *dep*, is associated with depolymerization of the capsular polymer (Uchida et al. 1993). Although the deduced amino acid sequence shows similarity to γ-glutamyl transpeptidases, the Dep protein, of 51.4 kDa, has no such activity. Dep appears to be an enzyme that catalyzes the hydrolysis of the poly-γ-D-glutamic acid capsule, controlling the size of the poly-glutamate capsule.

It would now be of great value to correlate the genetic information, which has accumulated concerning *B. anthracis* capsule synthetic enzymes, and the biochemical reactions, which have been described for *B. licheniformis*, and which may be identical to those in *B. anthracis*.

Furthermore, the specific components, if they exist, or specific mechanisms that ensure the capsule adhesion to the bacteria will have to be elucidated.

6 Role of Capsule and S-Layer

The capsule surrounds the bacilli found in animals infected by a virulent strain, indicating that it is synthesized in vivo (Cromartie et al. 1946a, b; Roth et al. 1960; Roth and Williams 1964). Furthermore, strains that do not synthesize capsule display an extremely attenuated pathogenicity, the capsule being a major virulence factor (Preisz 1909). For example, the LD_{50} in mice can be reduced by as much as 4 logs by the loss of the capsule (Welkos 1991). The contribution of capsule to pathogenicity is due to it enabling the bacteria to evade the host immune defenses and provoke septicemia. *B. anthracis* capsule inhibits phagocytosis (Preisz 1909; Zwartouw and Smith 1956; Makino et al. 1989). Furthermore, it is a monotonous linear polymer that is only very weakly immunogenic (Goodman and Nitecki 1967; Roelants et al. 1969). It has also been shown that polymers of D-isomers are far less immunogenic than those of L-amino acid residues (Maurer 1965; Parker et al. 1965). The characteristics of *B. anthracis* capsule therefore are not those favoring an immune response.

When capsule and S-layer are present, the capsule is the outermost element (Figs. 4, 6). In its presence, the cell surface is inaccessible to antibodies; no immunolabeling is observed with the anti-galactose/*N*-acetylglucosamine polysaccharide or with the anti-EA1 or anti-Sap antibodies (Ezzell and Abshire 1996; Mesnage et al. 1998). The S-layer components EA1 and Sap are able to form structured surface arrays under the capsule. However, the presence of an S-layer is not required for a normal capsulation of *B. anthracis* bacilli. This suggests that the capsule is anchored either to the peptidoglycan-containing sacculus or to the cytoplasmic membrane, independently of the S-layer proteins. Nevertheless, the S-layer may modify the fine structure of the capsule.

The role of the capsule in vivo is clear, but, mainly because of the independence of the two structures and the architecture of the surface components, that of the S-layer is not. However, the resources the bacterium devotes to their synthesis are such that it is hard to imagine that they have no role. Because of its ability to cause disseminated disease, the interaction

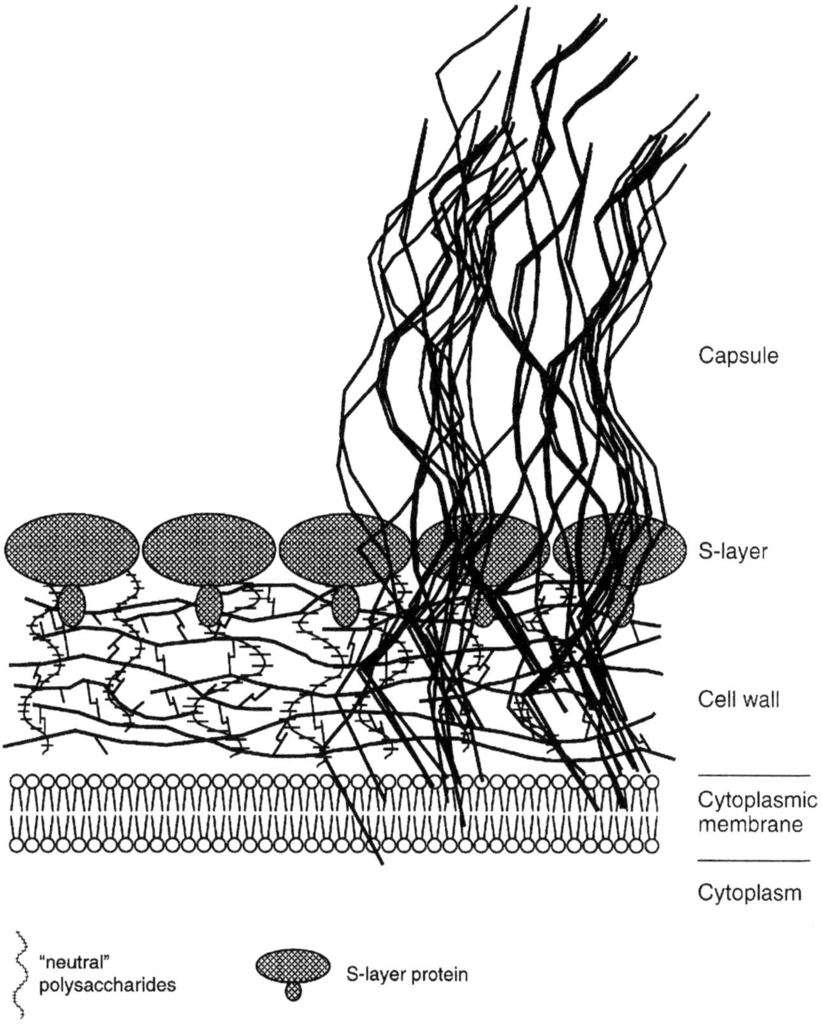

Fig. 6. Schematic representation of the cell envelope organization of *B. anthracis*, in the absence and in the presence of the capsule (*left*- and *right-hand* side of the figure, respectively)

of *B. anthracis* with phagocytic cells is important. The contribution of the surface structures to resistance to innate alternative complement pathway-mediated defenses and to complement binding has been studied (Ray et al. 1998). A strain synthesizing both capsule and S-layer proteins is the most resistant, whereas one displaying neither structure is the most sensitive to binding of the C3 component of complement. Strains having only one of these structures are slightly more sensitive than the parental strain. In the presence of human blood, the parental strain was the most resistant and strains possessing none of these structures or Sap only, were the most sensitive. Those with the capsule or EA1 had an intermediate resistance. Capsule and S-layer therefore seem to have a cumulative effect for resistance to complement pathway-mediated defenses, probably with Sap and EA1 having different roles. This could be due to differences in symmetry between the 2-dimensional crystals, or in localization at the bacterial surface, or in time of appearance. Structural and regulatory studies are required to resolve this issue. It would be valuable to understand how the complex *B. anthracis* surface appears in vivo immediately after the beginning of germination, during outgrowth, and during elongation of the bacilli. The outgrowth efficiency and timing vary in vitro, depending on the medium used. The capsule appears to emerge from spores as blebs that enlarge and coalesce, forming a continuous layer (Ezzell and Abshire 1996). The capsule may be, at any given moment or in some surface regions, not perfectly continuous, and the S-layer would then be the outermost structure.

7
Perspectives

Many questions remain concerning the surface structures of *B. anthracis*. Some have been highlighted in this review. Even the capsule, one of the two major virulence factors, is still not fully characterized. *B. anthracis*-specific surface structures should certainly be studied more thoroughly. Because of the renewed interest in this bacterium, genomic knowledge is rapidly progressing. pXO2, the plasmid encoding capsule synthetic activity, and pXO1 have been sequenced (accession numbers AF188935 and AF065404, respectively; Okinaka et al. 1999). The chromosome sequence is nearing completion (www.tigr.org), and DNA arrays and proteomics will soon make a large contribution. Therefore, many tools will be available, helping scientists in the field to progress quickly. Our growing understanding of

B. anthracis and the many genetic tools that have been developed over the last 10 years for this species allow it to be used as a model for mechanisms shared with other prokaryotes, for example, the SLH-anchoring mechanism. The limiting steps might now become biochemistry and structural biology. Finally, deciphering the *B. anthracis* surface structures should help understand the physiopathology of anthrax and help develop tools to fight this and other diseases caused by extracellular bacteria.

Acknowledgements. The authors thank M. Mock for her constant interest in the work on the *B. anthracis* surface and for her critical reading of this manuscript. We thank TIGR for making available the incomplete *Bacillus anthracis* genome sequence and particularly T. Read for specific analysis. S.M. was funded by the Ministère de l'Enseignement Supérieur et de la Recherche and by a "Bourse de la Fondation Roux."

References

Ascoli A (1911) Die Präzipitindiagnose bei Milzbrand. Zentralbl Bakt Paras Infekt Krank I orig 58:63–69

Ashiuchi M, Soda K, Misono H (1999) A poly-γ-glutamate synthetic system of *Bacillus subtilis* IFO 3336: gene cloning and biochemical analysis of poly-γ-glutamate produced by *Escherichia coli* clone cells. Biochem Biophys Res Commun 263:6–12

Atrih A, Zollner P, Allmaier G, Williamson MP, Foster SJ (1998) Peptidoglycan structural dynamics during germination of *Bacillus subtilis* 168 endospores. J Bacteriol 180:4603–4612

Avakyan AA, Katz LN, Levina KN, Pavlova IB (1965) Structure and composition of the *Bacillus anthracis* capsule. J Bacteriol 90:1082–1095

Bail O (1915) Veränderung der Bakterien in Tierkörper. Ueber die Korrelation zwischen Kapselbildung Sporenbildung und Infektiosität des Milzbrandbazillus. Zentralbl Bakt Paras Infekt Krank I orig 75:159–173

Beveridge TJ, Graham LL (1991) Surface layers of bacteria. Microbiol Rev 55:684–705

Bishop DG, Rutberg L, Samuelson B (1967) The chemical composition of the cytoplasmic membrane of *Bacillus subtilis*. Eur J Biochem 2:448–453

Brückner V, Kovacs J (1953) Structure of poly-D-glutamic acid isolated from capsulated strains of *Bacillus anthracis*. Nature 172:508

Burger M (1950) Anthrax polysaccharides. In: Thomas CC (ed) Bacterial Polysaccharides Springfield, USA, pp 121–134

Chauvaux S, Matuschek M, Beguin P (1999) Distinct affinity of binding sites for S-layer homologous domains in *Clostridium thermocellum* and *Bacillus anthracis* cell envelopes. J Bacteriol 181:2455–2458

Cromartie WJ, Bloom WL, Watson DW (1946a) Studies on infection with *Bacillus anthracis*. I. A histopathological study of skin lesions produced by *Bacillus anthracis* in susceptible and resistant animal species. J Infect Dis 80:1–13

Cromartie WJ, Watson DW, Bloom WL, Heckly RJ (1946b) Studies on infection with *Bacillus anthracis*. II. The immunological and tissue damaging properties of extracts prepared from lesions of *Bacillus anthracis* infection. J Infect Dis 80: 14–27

De Mendoza D, Farias R (1988) Effects of fatty acid supplementation on membrane fluidity in microorganisms. In: Aloia RC, Curtain CC, Gordon LM (eds) Physiological Regulation of Membrane Fluidity. Alan R. Liss, Inc. New York, Vol 3, pp 119–149

De Mendoza D, Grau R, Cronan Jr. JE (1993) Biosynthesis and function of membrane lipids. In: Sonenshein AL, Hoch JA, Losick R (eds) *Bacillus subtilis* and other gram-positive bacteria. American Society for Microbiology Washington, DC, pp 411–421

Doyle RJ, Koch AL (1987) The functions of autolysins in the growth and division of *Bacillus subtilis*. Crit Rev Microbiol 15:169–222

Eastin JD, Thorne CB (1963) Carbon dioxide fixation in *Bacillus anthracis*. J Bacteriol 85:410–417

Ekwunife FS, Singh J, Taylor KG, Doyle RJ (1991) Isolation and purification of cell wall polysaccharide of *Bacillus anthracis* (Δ Sterne). FEMS Microbiol Lett 82:257–262

Ellwood DC, Tempest DW (1972) Effects of environment on bacterial wall content and composition. Adv Microbiol Physiol 7:83–117

Etienne-Toumelin I, Sirard J-C, Duflot E, Mock M, Fouet A (1995) Characterization of the *Bacillus anthracis* S-layer: cloning and sequencing of the structural gene. J Bacteriol 177:614–620

Ezzell Jr. JW, Abshire TG (1988) Immunological analysis of cell-associated antigens of *Bacillus anthracis*. Infect Immun 56:349–356

Ezzell Jr. JW, Abshire TG, Little SF, Lidgarding BC, Brown C (1990) Identification of *Bacillus anthracis* by using monoclonal antibody to cell wall galactose-*N*-acetylglucosamine polysaccharide. J Clin Microbiol 28:223–231

Ezzell JW, Abshire TG (1996) Encapsulation of *Bacillus anthracis* spores and spore identification. In: Turnbull, PCB (ed), Proceedings of the International Workshop on Anthrax. Salisbury Medical Bulletin, Special Supplement n° 87, p. 42

Fox A, Black GE, Fox K, Rostovtseva S (1993) Determination of carbohydrate profiles of *Bacillus anthracis* and *Bacillus cereus* including identification of *O*-methyl methylpentoses by using gas chromatography-mass spectrometry. J Clin Microbiol 31:887–894

Gardner JM, Troy FA (1979) Chemistry and biosynthesis of the poly (γ-D-glutamyl) capsule in *Bacillus licheniformis*. Activation, racemization, and polymerization of glutamic acid by a membranous polyglutamyl synthetase complex. J Biol Chem 254:6262–6269

Gerhardt P (1967) Cytology of *Bacillus anthracis*. Fed Proc 26:1504–1517

Ghuysen J-M (1968) Use of bacteriolytic enzymes in determination of wall structure and their role in cell metabolism. Bacteriol Rev 32:425–464

Goodman JW, Nitecki DE (1967) Studies on the relation of a prior immune response to immunogenicity. Immunology 13:577–583

Graham LL, Beveridge TJ (1994) Structural differentiation of the *Bacillus subtilis* 168 cell wall. J Bacteriol 176:1413–1421

Green BD, Battisti L, Koehler TM, Thorne CB, Ivins BE (1985) Demonstration of a capsule plasmid in *Bacillus anthracis*. Infect Immun 49:291–297

Guffanti AA, Clejan S, Falk LH, Hicks DB, Krulwich TA (1987) Isolation and characterization of uncoupler resistant mutants of *Bacillus subtilis*. J Bacteriol 169:4479–4485

Haldenwang WG (1995) The sigma factors of *Bacillus subtilis*. Microbiol Rev 59:1–30

Hanby WE, Rydon HN (1946) The capsular susbtance of *Bacillus anthracis*. Biochem J 40:297–309

Hancock IC (1983) Activation and inactivation of secondary wall polymers in *Bacillus subtilis* W23. Arch Microbiol 134:222–226

Hancock IC (1997) Bacterial cell surface carbohydrates: structure and assembly. Biochem Soc Trans 25:183–187

Holt SC, Leadbetter ER (1969) Comparative ultrastructure of selected aerobic spore-forming bacteria: a freeze-etching study. Bacteriol Rev 33:346–378

Huang X, Helmann JD (1998) Identification of target promoters for the *Bacillus subtilis* σ^X factor using a consensus-directed search. J Mol Biol 279:165–173

Ivánovics G, Brückner V (1937a) Notiz zu unserer Mitteilung: chemische und immunologische Studien über den Mechanismus der Milzbrandinfektion und Immunität. Zeitschr Immunitätsf 91:175–176

Ivánovics G, Brückner V (1937b) Chemische und immunologische Studien über den Mechanismus der Milzbrandinfektion und Immunität. Zeitschr Immunitätsf 90:304–318

Iwasaki H, Shimada A, Yokoyama K, Ito E (1989) Structure and glycosylation of lipoteichoic acids in *Bacillus* strains. J Bacteriol 171:424–429

Jolliffe LK, Doyle RJ, Streips UN (1981) The energized membrane and cellular autolysis in *Bacillus subtilis*. Cell 25:753–763

Kaneda T (1991) Iso- and anteiso-fatty acids in bacteria: biosynthesis, function, and taxonomic significance. Microbiol Rev 55:288–302

Kawata T, Takeoka A, Takumi K, Masuda K (1984) Demonstration and preliminary characterization of a regular array in the cell wall of *Clostridium difficile*. FEMS Microbiol Lett 24:323–328

Koch AL, Doyle RJ (1985) Inside-to-outside growth and turnover of the wall of gram-positive rods. J Theor Biol 117:137–157

König H, Niemetz R (1997) Polyglutamate surface polypeptides in Bacteria and Archae. FEMS Microbiol Rev 20:36–39

Kotiranta A, Haapasalo M, Kari K, Kerosuo E, Olsen I, Sorsa T, Meurman JH, Lounatmaa K (1998) Surface structure, hydrophobicity, phagocytosis, and adherence to matrix proteins of *Bacillus cereus* cells with and without the crystalline surface protein layer. Infect Immun 66:4895–4902

Kramar E (1922) Untersuchungen über die chemische Beschaffenheit der Kapselsubstanz einiger Kapselbakterien. Centralbl f Bakt I Abt Originale 87:401–406

Kunst F, Ogasawara N, Moszer I, Albertini AM, Alloni G, Azevedo V, Bertero MG, Bessieres P, Bolotin A, Borchert S, Borris R, Boursier L, Brans A, Braun M, Brignell SC, Bron S, Brouillet S, Bruschi CV, Caldwell B, Capuano V, Carter NM, Choi SK, Codani JJ, Connerton IF, Danchin A (1997) The complete genome sequence of the gram-positive bacterium *Bacillus subtilis*. Nature 390:237–238

Kuroda A, Asami Y, Sekiguchi J (1993) Molecular cloning of a sporulation-specific cell wall hydrolase gene of *Bacillus subtilis.* J Bacteriol 175:6260–6268

Lawrence D, Heitefuss S, Seifert HS (1991) Differentiation of *Bacillus anthracis* from *Bacillus cereus* by gas chromatographic whole-cell fatty acid analysis. J Clin Microbiol 29:1508–1512

Lemaire M, Ohayon H, Gounon P, Fujino T, Béguin P (1995) OlpB, a new outer layer protein of *Clostridium thermocellum*, and binding of its S-layer-like domains to components of the cell envelope. J Bacteriol 177:2451–2459

Lennarz WJ (1970) Bacterial lipids. In: Wakil JJ (ed) Lipid Metabolism. Academic Press, Inc. New York

Leonard CG, Housewright RD (1963) Polyglutamic acid synthesis by cell-free extracts of *Bacillus licheniformis.* Biochim Biophys Acta 73:530–532

Lindeque PM, Turnbull PC (1994) Ecology and epidemiology of anthrax in the Etosha National Park, Namibia. Onderstepoort J Vet Res 61:71–83

Lupas A, Engelhardt H, Peters J, Santarius U, Volker S, Baumeister W (1994) Domain structure of the *Acetogenium kivui* surface layer revealed by electron crystallography and sequence analysis. J Bacteriol 176:1224–1233

Makino SI, Uchida I, Terakado N, Sasakawa C, Yoshikawa M (1989) Molecular characterization and protein analysis of the *cap* region, which is essential for encapsulation in *Bacillus anthracis.* J Bacteriol 171:722–730

Maurer PH (1965) Antigenicity of polypeptides (poly alpha amino acids). XIII. Immunological studies with synthetic polymers containing only D- or D- and L-α-amino acids. J Exp Med 121:339–349

Merad T, Archibald AR, Hancock IC, Harwood CR, Hobot JA (1989) Cell wall assembly in *Bacillus subtilis*: visualization of old and new wall material by electron microscopic examination of samples stained selectively for teichoic acid and teichuronic acid. J Gen Microbiol 135:645–655

Mesnage S, Fontaine T, Mignot T, Delepierre M, Mock M, and Fouet A (2000). Bacterial SLH-domain proteins are non-covalently anchored to the cell surface via a conserved mechanism involving wall-polysaccharide pyruvylation. EMBO J *19*: 4473–4484

Mesnage S, Tosi Couture E, Mock M, Fouet A (1999a) The S-layer homology domain as a means for anchoring heterologous proteins on the cell surface of *Bacillus anthracis.* J Appl Microbiol 87:256–260

Mesnage S, Tosi-Couture E, Gounon P, Mock M, Fouet A (1998) The capsule and S-layer: two independent and yet compatible macromolecular structures in *Bacillus anthracis.* J Bacteriol 180:52–58

Mesnage S, Tosi-Couture E, Mock M, Gounon P, Fouet A (1997) Molecular characterization of the *Bacillus anthracis* main S-layer component: evidence that it is the major cell-associated antigen. Mol Microbiol 23:1147–1155

Mesnage S, Weber-Levy M, Haustant M, Mock M, Fouet A (1999b) Cell surface-exposed tetanus toxin fragment C produced by recombinant *Bacillus anthracis* protects against tetanus toxin. Infect Immun 67:4847–4850

Messner P, Sleytr UB (1992) Crystalline bacterial cell-surface layers. Adv Microb Physiol 33:212–275

Meynell E, Meynell GG (1964) The roles of serum and carbon dioxide in capsule formation by *Bacillus anthracis.* J Gen Microbiol 34:153–164

Meynell GG, Meynell E (1966) The biosynthesis of poly D-glutamic acid, the capsular material of *Bacillus anthracis.* J Gen Microbiol 43:119–138

Mignot T, Mesnage S, Couture-Tosi E, Mock M, Fouet A (2002) Developmental switch of S-layer protein synthesis in Bacillus anthracis. Mol Microbiol 43:1615–1627

Molnár J, Prágai B (1971) Attempts to detect the presence of teichoic acid in *Bacillus anthracis.* Acta Microbiol Acad Sci Hung 18:105–108

Okinaka RT, Cloud K, Hampton O, Hoffmaster AR, Hill KK, Keim P, Koehler TM, Lamke G, Kumano S, Mahillon J, Manter D, Martinez Y, Ricke D, Svensson R, Jackson PJ (1999) Sequence and organization of pXO1, the large *Bacillus anthracis* plasmid harboring the anthrax toxin genes. J Bacteriol 181: 6509–6515

Olabarría G, Carrascosa JL, de Pedro MA, Berenguer J (1996) A conserved motif in S-layer proteins is involved in peptidoglycan binding in *Thermus thermophilus.* J Bacteriol 178:4765–4772

Parker CW, Thiel JA, Mitchell S (1965) The immunogenicity of hapten-polylysine conjugates. J Immunol 94:289–294

Pooley HM (1976) Layered distribution, according to age, within the cell wall of *Bacillus subtilis.* J Bacteriol 125:1139–1147

Preisz H (1909) Experimentelle Studien über Virulenz, Empfänglichkeit und Immunität beim Milzbrand. Zeitschr Immunitätsf 5:341–452

Quinn CP, Turnbull PCB (1998) Anthrax. In: Hausler Jr WJ, Sussman M (eds) Microbiology and Microbial Infections: Bacterial Infections. Topley & Wilson's, Ninth edition London, Sydney, Auckland, Vol 3, pp 799–818

Ray KC, Mesnage S, Washburn R, Mock M, Fouet A, Blaser M (1998) Complement binding to *Bacillus anthracis* mutants lacking surface structures. Abstracts Book Poster 98th General Meeting. American Society for Microbiology Atlanta, Georgia, USA, pp B-418

Record BR, Wallis RG (1956) Physicochemical examination of polyglutamic acid from *Bacillus anthracis* grown in vivo. Biochem J 63:443–447

Ries W, Hotzy C, Schocher I, Sleytr UB, Sára M (1997) Evidence that the N-terminal part of the S-layer protein from *Bacillus stearothermophilus* pv72/p2 recognizes a secondary cell wall polymer. J Bacteriol 179:3892–3898

Roelants GE, Senyk G, Goodman JW (1969) Immunochemical studies on the poly-γ-D-glutamyl capsule of *Bacillus anthracis.* V. The in vivo fate and distribution in rabbits of the polypeptide in immunogenic and nonimmunogenic forms. Israel J Med Sci 5:196–208

Roth IL, Lewis J, CWL, Williams RP (1960) Electron microscope study of *Bacillus anthracis* in mouse spleen. J Bacteriol 80:772–782

Roth IL, Williams RP (1964) Nature of the cytopathic area surrounding virulent cells of *Bacillus anthracis* in mouse spleen. J Bacteriol 88:523–530

Salton MRJ (1994) The bacterial cell envelope – a historical perspective. In: Ghuysen J-M, Hakenbeck R (eds.) The Bacterial Cell Wall. Elsevier Science B.V. Amsterdam, The Netherlands, Vol 27, pp 1–22

Sára M, Kuen B, Mayer HF, Mandl F, Schuster KC, Sleytr UB (1996) Dynamics in oxygen-induced changes in S-layer protein synthesis from *Bacillus stearothermophilus* PV72 and the S-layer-deficient variant T5 in continuous culture and studies of the cell wall composition. J Bacteriol 178:2108–2117

Schleifer KH, Kandler O (1972) Peptidoglycan types of bacterial cell walls and their taxonomic implications. Bacteriol Rev 36:407–477

Sekiguchi J, Akeo K, Yamamoto H, Khasanov FK, Alonso JC, Kuroda A (1995) Nucleotide sequence and regulation of a new putative cell wall hydrolase gene, *cwlD*, which affects germination in *Bacillus subtilis*. J Bacteriol 177:5582–5589

Shockman GD, Barrett JF (1983) Structure, function and assembly of cell walls of gram-positive bacteria. Ann Rev Microbiol 37:501–527

Shockman GD, Höltje J-V (1994) Microbial peptidoglycan (murein) hydrolases. In: Ghuysen J-M, Hakenbeck R (eds) Bacterial Cell Wall. Elsevier Science B.V. Amsterdam, The Netherlands, Vol 27, pp 131–166

Simonen M, Palva I (1993) Protein secretion in *Bacillus* species. Microbiol Rev 57: 109–137

Sleytr UB, Messner P (1983) Crystalline surface layers on bacteria. Ann Rev Microbiol 37:311–339

Sleytr UB, Messner P, Pum D, Sara M (1993) Crystalline bacterial cell surface layers. Mol Microbiol 10:911–916

Sleytr UB, Messner P, Pum D, Sara M (1996) Occurrence, location, ultrastructure and morphogenesis of S-Layers. In: Sleytr UW, Messner P, Pum D, Sara M (eds) Crystalline Bacterial Cell Surface Proteins. Academic Press New York, pp 5–33

Smith TJ, Blackman SA, Foster SJ (1996) Peptidoglycan hydrolases of *Bacillus subtilis* 168. Microb Drug Resist 2:113–118

Soldo B, Lazarevic V, Pagni M, Karamata D (1999) Teichuronic acid operon of *Bacillus subtilis* 168. Mol Microbiol 31:795–805

Takumi K, Koga T, Oka T, Endo Y (1991) Self-assembly, adhesion, and chemical properties of tetragonarly arrayed S-layer proteins of *Clostridium*. J Gen Appl Microbiol 37:455–465

Thorne CB (1956) Capsule formation and glutamyl polypeptide synthesis by *Bacillus anthracis* and *Bacillus subtilis*. In: Spooner ETC, Stocker BAD (eds) Bacterial Anatomy. Cambridge University Press Cambridge, pp 68–80

Thorne CB (1993) *Bacillus anthracis*. In: Sonenshein AL, Hoch JA, Losick R (eds) *Bacillus subtilis* and other Gram-positive Bacteria. American Society for Microbiology Washington, DC, pp 113–124

Thorne CB, Leonard CG (1958) Isolation of D- and L-glutamyl polypeptides from culture filtrates of *Bacillus subtilis*. J Biol Chem 233:1109–1112

Tomcsik J (1956) Bacterial capsules and their relation to the cell wall. In: Spooner ETC, Stocker BAD (eds.) Bacterial Anatomy. Cambridge University Press Cambridge, pp 41–67

Tomcsik J, Szongott H (1933) Ueber ein spezifisches Protein der Kapsel des Milzbrandbazillus. Zeitschr Immunitätsf 78:86–99

Troy FA (1973a) Chemistry and biosynthesis of the poly (γ-D-glutamyl) capsule in *Bacillus licheniformis*. I. Properties of the membrane mediated biosynthetic reaction. J Biol Chem 248:305–315

Troy FA (1973b) Chemistry and biosynthesis of the poly (γ-D-glutamyl) capsule in *Bacillus licheniformis*. II. Characterization and structural properties of the enzymatically synthesis polymer. J Biol Chem 248:316–324

Tsuboi A, Tsukagoshi N, Udaka S (1982) Reassembly in vitro of hexagonal surface arrays in a protein-producing bacterium, *Bacillus brevis* 47. J Bacteriol 151:1485–1497

Uchida I, Makino S, Sasakawa C, Yoshikawa M, Sugimoto C, Terakado N (1993) Identification of a novel gene, *dep*, associated with depolymerization of the capsular polymer in *Bacillus anthracis*. Mol Microbiol 9:487–496

Uchida I, Sekizaki T, Hashimoto K, Terakado N (1985) Association of the encapsulation of *Bacillus anthracis* with a 60-megadalton plasmid. J Gen Microbiol 131: 363–367

Vanden Boom T, Cronan Jr. JE (1989) Genetics and regulation of bacterial lipid metabolism. Annu Rev Microbiol 43:317–343

Welkos SL (1991) Plasmid-associated virulence factors of non-toxigenic (pXO1–) *Bacillus anthracis*. Microb Pathog 10:183–198

Zipperle Jr. GF, Ezzell Jr. J, Doyle RJ (1984) Glucosamine substitution and muramidase susceptibility in *Bacillus anthracis*. Can J Microbiol 30:553–559

Zwartouw HT, Smith H (1956) Polyglutamic acid from *Bacillus anthracis* grown in vivo: structure and aggressin activity. Biochem J 63:437–454

Chapter 6

Macrophage Interactions

C. Guidi-Rontani, M. Mock

Abstract. *B. anthracis* virulence is the sum of the contributions of factors involved in toxicity, growth and persistence in the host. Recent data has revealed that the interactions between *B. anthracis* and macrophage is central to the *B. anthracis* pathogenesis. This review presents and describes tactics by which *B. anthracis* not only overcomes and avoids macrophages but also perverts the host defense immune system and defense-related products to its advantage. The understanding of the complex network of such interactions is likely to allow new therapeutic and preventative strategies to be developed.

C. Guidi-Rontani, M. Mock
Unité Toxines et Pathogénie Bactériennes, CNRS URA 2172, Institut Pasteur, 28 rue du Dr. Roux, 75015 Paris, France, Email: rontani@pasteur.fr; mmock@pasteur.fr.

1 Introduction

When in 1905 METCHNIKOFF, using *Bacillus anthracis* as a model, identified the three main characteristics of the macrophage, diapedesis (KERR 1999), chemotaxis (BINDER et al. 1999), and phagocytosis (GREENBERG 1999) and thereby defined the macrophage cell, he was far from realizing that the interactions between these two partners would be central to the understanding of *B. anthracis* pathogenesis. *B. anthracis,* a Gram-positive, endospore-forming, aerobic rod-shaped bacterium, interacts with macrophages at various stages of the disease. Anthrax is a zoonosis to which most mammals are susceptible. Other species including reptiles and amphibians are also susceptible to varying degrees (STEPHEN 1981, 1986). During the past several years, there has been considerable research on the physiopathology of anthrax. However, our understanding of the cellular and molecular interactions between *B. anthracis* and host immune cells is far from complete, and many important questions remain. *B. anthracis* colonizes the host using a repertoire of virulence determinants, causing bacteremia and toxemia, the combination of which results in systemic anthrax. The major known *B. anthracis* virulence factors include cell surface-associated antiphagocytic poly-γ-D-glutamic acid capsule (GREEN et al. 1985), and two toxins, the edema (EdTx) and lethal (LeTx) toxins (BEALL et al. 1962; FRIEDLANDER 1986). Spore germination and outgrowth of vegetative bacilli are crucial steps enabling the bacteria to proliferate actively and to synthesize the virulence factors leading to a massive septicemia. The final phase of systemic anthrax is associated with onset of hypotension, shock-like symptoms, and sudden death resulting from a complex cascade of events.

For successful infection, a pathogen has to defeat and to survive the host immune system. To deal with this hostile and effective antimicrobial environment, *B. anthracis* avoids and even breaches specific cells including neutrophils and monocytes/macrophages, which play a key role in both clearance of the invading bacteria and production of antibacterial factors. In the absence of tight and coordinated regulation, the activities of these defense-related products involved in the eradication of invading microorganisms may lead to the destruction of host tissues (GALLIN and SNYDERMAN 1999). Recent insights into the modulation of the cytokines and the signaling pathway via *B. anthracis* have revealed much about the delicate underlying balance between the strategies used by *B. anthracis* to survive within a host and the concomitant efforts of the host to kill it.

This chapter presents and describes tactics by which *B. anthracis* not only overcomes and avoids macrophages, the protectors against bacterial infection, but also perverts the host defense immune system and defense-related products to its advantage.

2
Interaction of *B. anthracis* with the Macrophage

2.1
The Spore: An Intracellular Behavior

The discovery that anthrax organisms form spores was one of the significant events in the science of microbiology and disease (KOCH 1876). Anthrax was linked with endemic soil contamination long before *B. anthracis* was identified as the causative organism (DAVAINE 1863; KOCH 1876; PASTEUR 1877). Despite large-scale vaccination of cattle, eradication of *B. anthracis* is difficult because dormant spores persist for decades in the environment (spores of the genus *Bacillus* have a half-life of about 100 years; HALVORSON 1997), ensuring virtual perpetuity of the species in the soil (MILES et al 1988; DE VOS 1990). Temperature and humidity appear to have a large influence on the persistence of anthrax spores (DAVIES 1960). Nevertheless, the spores can resist and survive prolonged exposure to diverse stresses such as desiccation, solvents, and extremes in pH, temperature, pressure, and ultraviolet and ionizing radiation (GOULD 1977; RUSSELL 1990). Discovery of the spore's resistance led to obvious conclusions about its role in species survival and occulted its involvement in other processes, in particular, its contribution to anthrax pathogenesis. This contribution is evident from the frequent presence of spores when infection is initiated, whatever the infection route. More recently, because of their high resistance (ERRINGTON 1993; MANCHEE et al. 1981, 1990) *B. anthracis* spores have been perceived as potential weapons for bioterrorism (INGLESBY 1999).

2.1.1
Spore Ultrastructure

Dormant spores of *B. anthracis* have a relatively complex structural anatomy (Fig. 1). The mature spore is made up of two main zones, a refractile core and a dark integument composed of differentiated layers (GERHARDT 1967). The core, an undifferentiated electron-transparent area, consists of

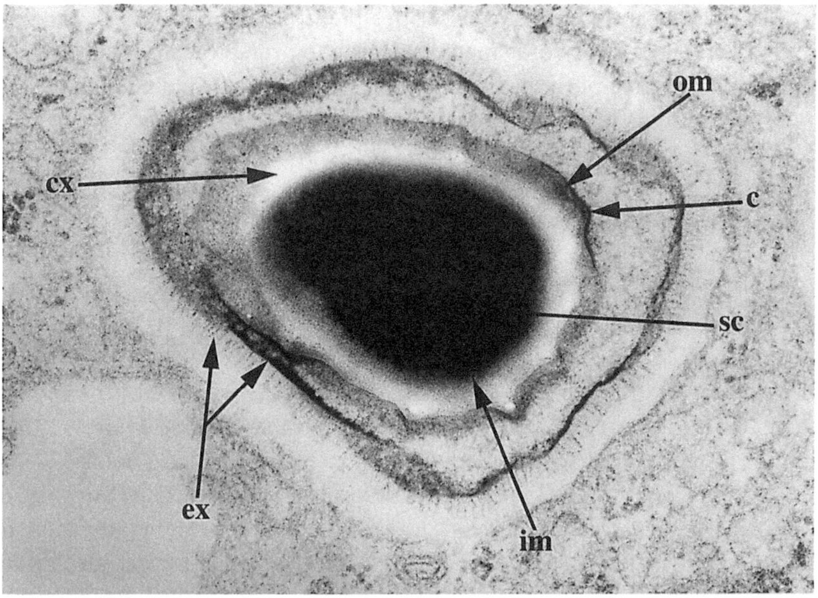

Fig. 1. Dormant spore of *Bacillus anthracis* within macrophage shown by transmission electron microscopy. Spores were sectioned and heavy metal stained. The main structural components of the spore are labeled: exosporium (*ex*); coat (*c*); outer membrane (*om*); cortex (*cx*); inner membrane (*im*); spore core (*sc*). The core consists of the cytoplasm and nucleoplasm enclosed by the inner membrane (Micrograph by H. Ohayon, Station Centrale de Microscopie Electronique, Institut Pasteur). × 146,000

the cytoplasm and nucleoplasm surrounded by the inner membrane and the outer membrane, both derived from mother cell membrane of opposing polarity. The inner membrane ultimately becomes the cytoplasmic membrane of the vegetative cell resulting from germination (Cleveland and Gilvarg 1975). A key structure in the survival of the organism is the cortex. This structure, a thick, electron-transparent layer located between these two membranes, is composed of dipicolinic acid and muropeptide polymer with a structure similar to that of the vegetative cell wall (Foster 1994). It is believed to be the main contributor to heat resistance. It also maintains the dormancy of the spore through contraction of the cortical mucopeptide so as to dehydrate the core (Murrell 1969). The coat, a thick, rigid, electron-opaque layer is a complex protein shell synthesized in the mother cell and assembled round the outer membrane of the forespore. This structure is not essential for dormancy or heat resistance but is important in the resistance of the spore to attack by enzymes such as lysozyme (MOIR and SMITH 1990).

The outermost integument of *B. anthracis* spores was discovered by DE BARY (1885) and named "exosporium" by FLÜGGE (1886). The exosporium is the primary physiological barrier between the spore and its environment and is the antigenic determinant of the spore (TOMCSIK et al. 1959). In contrast to other integument structures, the exosporium is biosynthesized de novo during sporogenesis (BECHTEL and BULLA 1976), and not by growth from a preexisting membrane, at the very beginning of cortex formation (OHYE and MURRELL 1973). Moreover, vegetative cells do not contain exosporium antigens (DESROSIER and LARA 1984). High-resolution electron microscopy revealed a surprisingly complex physical ultrastructure: the exosporium consists of a paracrystalline basal layer, 100 A thick, with a p6 hexagonal lattice structure (WELHRLI et al. 1980) and a hair-like outer layer with hairs 60 to 85 A in diameter and 180 to greater than 600 A in length, depending on the strain (Vollum and Sterne, respectively) (GERHARDT and RIBI 1964; HACHISUKA et al. 1966). The exosporium is composed of protein, lipid, and carbohydrate (MATZ et al. 1970; BEAMAN et al. 1971). However, the proteins that make up the structural framework have not been identified. Recently, exosporium-specific glycoproteins have been shown in *B. thuringiensis* (GARCIA-PATRONE and TANDECARZ 1995) and in *B. cereus* (CHARLTON et al. 1999). The function of the exosporium is unknown, and its contribution, if any, to the pathogenesis of *B. anthracis* remains to be demonstrated.

2.1.2 *Spore Germination*

B. anthracis can infect the host, leading to anthrax via intradermal inoculation, ingestion, or inhalation of spores (LAFORCE et al. 1969; FRIEDLANDER et al. 1993b; KLEIN et al. 1966). Among the different exposures leading to infection, the pulmonary form of anthrax causes the rapid progression of the disease and is always deadly (inhalational anthrax in humans is virtually 100% fatal) (BARNES 1947; FRITZ et al. 1995; ZAUCHA et al. 1998). As early as 1888 BUCHNER and co-workers found it possible to infect mice, guinea pigs, and rabbits by inhalation of clouds of anthrax spores. This was later confirmed by ENDERLEN (1889), who was able to infect sheep in the same manner. These important early studies demonstrated that anthrax infection could be established through the lung.

Between 5×10^4 and 1×10^5 spores are required to infect rabbits by intranasal instillation; the 50% aerosol lethal dose (LD_{50}) for *B. anthracis* spores of the virulent Ames strain in the rabbit model is 1.05×10^5 colony-forming units (CFU) (Zaucha et al. 1998).

Histopathological studies of fatally infected mice, guinea pigs, monkeys (Fritz et al. 1995), rabbits (Zaucha et al. 1998), and sheep indicate that respiratory exposure to anthrax spores results in a general infection rather than in a true pulmonary disease. The lung serves only as a point of invasion, and the organism is transported elsewhere to sites where it causes the bacillemia characteristic of fatal anthrax infections. The observations (Gleiser et al. 1963; Abramova et al. 1993) that some monkeys and sheep infected by inhalation may have lung mites and anthrax-related pneumonia are thought to result from lesions in the lungs before exposure to anthrax spores (Fritz et al. 1995).

In vitro and in vivo experiments have demonstrated that, once inhaled, spores reach the respiratory bronchioles and alveoli; most are subject to rapid and efficient phagocytosis by alveolar macrophages via recruitment of F-actin (Ross 1957; Shafa et al. 1966; Guidi-Rontani et al. 1999a). This actin reorganization indicated that the receptors for the Fc portion of IgG (FcRs) (Greenberg et al. 1991) are the mediators of the phagocytosis of *B. anthracis* spore via Rac1 and Cdc42 (Caron and Hall 1998). The spore-bearing macrophages migrate along the lymphatic channels to the regional lymph nodes, to local mediastinal lymph nodes (Ross 1957; Lincoln et al. 1965), and from there to the blood stream. Germination therefore appears to be essential for the establishment of anthrax disease.

Early observations suggested that *B. anthracis* spores could germinate within alveolar macrophages, but the tools to proceed further were not then available (Ross 1957; Shafa et al. 1966). Modern high-resolution visualization techniques, allowing the identification of molecular components within cellular compartments, in association with analysis of cells freshly isolated from infected animals, have made it possible to demonstrate the efficient germination of *B. anthracis* spores within macrophages, for example, alveolar macrophages (Guidi-Rontani et al. 1999a). The importance of favorable internal conditions for spore germination in the establishment of anthrax was clearly demonstrated by Hachisuka (1969), who used the peritoneal cavity of rats as a model. Hachisuka proposed that factors associated with early steps of infection, before the appearance of vegetative cells, determine natural resistance or sensitivity to anthrax. The germination process, which is an irreversible series of degradative reactions that results in the breaking of spore dormancy, is still poorly understood (Foster and Johnstone 1990). L-Alanine, DL-tyrosine, and adenosine are effective germination inducers (HILLS 1949), and L-alanine appears to be the major germination-inducing chemical in serum (Titball and Manchee 1987).

Recently, the first germination operon (*gerX*) of *B. anthracis* was identified (Guidi-Rontani et al. 1999b). The *gerX*-encoded proteins (GerXB, GerXA and GerXC) may be virulence factors and contribute to the pathogenesis of *B. anthracis* (Guidi-Rontani et al. 1999b) by constituting a specific receptor or antennae (Yasuda and Tochikubo 1984). It is clear that the germination rate may have a crucial effect on the outcome of the infection. However, the establishment of anthrax disease may require not only the rapid emergence of the vegetative form but also that this occurs in a favorable niche. Indeed, *B. anthracis* spores may possess a unique system for detecting specific germinants within macrophage in the host, but such putative germinants remain to be identified. This identification may allow the design of drugs to inactivate *B. anthracis* targets essential for the early steps of the infection. The *gerX* locus is the only germination operon known that is located on a virulence plasmid. Interestingly, the *gerX* operon maps to the large toxin-encoding region of 40 kb, flanked by two inverted repeat elements of pXO1 (185 kb) (Hornung and Thorne; EMBL accession nos. U30715 and U30713). This region also harbors the structural genes, *pagA, lef, cya, atxA*, and *pagR* encoding the three toxin components (Leppla 1991), their transcriptional activator AtxA (Uchida et al. 1993; Koehler et al. 1994), and the transcriptional repressor of *pagA* and *atxA*, respectively (Hoffmaster and Koehler 1999). This fragment with virulence-associated functions also harbors two Tn1546-related elements (Arthur et al. 1993), one resolvase-like and one transposase-like (Guidi-Rontani et al; GenBank accession no. AF150965). These results allowed the pXO1 region to be proposed as the first pathogenicity island of *B. anthracis* (Guidi-Rontani et al. 1999b; Okinaka et al. 1999).

Another germination operon (*gerY*) on the *B. anthracis* chromosome was recently identified (Guidi-Rontani et al; GenBank accession no. AF182371). Data from the *B. anthracis* genome sequencing program at TIGR indicate that *B. anthracis* contains at least five loci encoding germination-like proteins (T. Read, personal communication). Germination operons located on the chromosome were expected because *B. anthracis* strains lacking pXO1 and pXO2 are able to germinate in vitro (Cataldi et al. 1990).

B. anthracis, like *B. subtilis*, probably possesses several germinant-specific receptors, enabling the spore to respond to different stimuli. Various germinant systems have been described in the genus *Bacillus*. In *B. subtilis*, the *gerA* operon (Zuberi et al. 1985, 1987) is required for the L-alanine response and the *gerB* (Corfe et al. 1994) and *gerK* (Irie et al. 1996) operons for the L-asparagine, glucose, fructose, and potassium ion responses. The *gerI* locus (Clements and Moir 1998) is required for inosine germination in *B. cereus*. Each of these germination pathways, stimulated by diverse triggering events, subsequently converges in the later stages of germination (Moir and Smith 1990).

The putative germination pathways imply spatial and functional interaction of *ger*-encoded proteins (McCann et al. 1996), but the exact functions of the various Ger proteins in the genus *Bacillus* are still unknown. It is likely that any germinant-sensing complex would require membrane-associated proteins such as an integral transmembrane protein and a highly hydrophobic protein with membrane-spanning helices. A lipoprotein, such as homologs of GerAC, is probably attached to the membrane of the forespore and may expose its hydrophilic domains to the environment so as to be accessible to the germinant. The ultrastructural locations of *ger*-encoded proteins within the spore lead to conflicting conclusions about the subcellular localization of the germinant-receptors. In light of the expression of the *gerA* locus in space and time and the observation that the spore is constructed in a stepwise fashion, from both the outside in and from the inside out, Moir and collaborators proposed that the inner spore membrane is the final localization (Feavers et al. 1990; Moir et al. 1994). In contrast, Yasuda and collaborators revealed by transmission immunoelectron microscopy and scanning immunoelectron microscopy that the *B. subtilis* GerAA, GerAB, and GerAC proteins are abundant in the boundary region between the cortex and the spore coat (Sakae et al. 1995; Yasuda et al. 1996).

New technology such as confocal scanning laser microscopy can be used to study host macrophage-pathogen interactions in single cells and to analyze and dissect the contribution of the alveolar macrophages during the first stage of infection. *B. anthracis* has to circumvent the oxidative burst resulting from microbicidal NADPH-oxidase activation, detoxifying and eliminating internally generated reactive oxygen species. NADPH oxidase, which is present in the membrane of the phagosome, catalyzes the reduction of molecular oxygen to superoxide anion (O_2^-) by oxidation of NADPH. The O_2^- is subsequently converted to other reactive oxygen species, including hydrogen peroxide (H_2O_2), peroxynitrite ($OONO^-$), and hypochlorous acid (HOCl) (HAMPTON et al. 1998). It remains to be determined whether superoxide dismutase, catalase, and alkyl hydroperoxide reductase (BEAMAN and BEAMAN 1984) are produced by *B. anthracis*.

The germination of *B. anthracis* within the mouse alveolar macrophage is colocalized with CD107-positive phagosomes (GUIDI-RONTANI et al. 1999a). *B. anthracis* spores or vegetative cells in the phagolysosome, an extremely effective antimicrobial environment, must face acidification of the phagolysosome and deal with the released lysosomal acid hydrolases. The mechanisms by which *B. anthracis* escapes destruction in this harsh environment have not been identified. A number of pathogens enter the host cell cytoplasm to survive and multiply (MOULDER 1985). Alternatively, bacteria may delay and reduce phagolysosome acidification. This is the approach taken by *Salmonella typhimurium* (ALPUCHE ARANDA et al. 1993) and *Histoplasma capsulatum* (EISSENBERG et al. 1993). Bacteria such as the acidophilic bacterium *Coxiella burnetii* have an absolute requirement for low pH to activate their metabolism (HACKSTADT 1983; THOMPSON and WILLIAMS 1991).

It is possible that changes in pH act as a stimulus for *B. anthracis* spores, leading to the transcription and translation of the acid-resistance loci necessary for intracellular survival. Although metabolically inert, the dormant spores are not inactive enzymologically. Several proteins associated with the spore exosporium have been described. An alanine racemase, which converts L-alanine to a mixture of L- and D-alanine, and an adenosine deaminase have been described in spores of *B. cereus* (BERGER and MARR 1960). A zinc metalloprotease homolog of immune inhibitor A (InA), found in *B. thuringiensis* and thought to specifically degrade two proteins of the insect immune system (DALHAMMAR and STEINER 1984), has been described in *B. anthracis* and *B.cereus*. A homolog of the *B. subtilis* RocA (1-pyrroline-5-carboxylate dehydrogenase) has been found in *B. cereus* (CHARLTON et al. 1999). Although the role of an alanine racemase in germination is evident, the role of these other enzymes is more obscure. However, it is not clear whether these proteins are true components of the exosporium or proteins from spore or mother cell lysis that have been adsorbed onto the exosporium.

To exploit niches within the host efficiently, *B. anthracis* must adapt its metabolic processes appropriately. Macrophages are a highly versatile cell type with an impressive repertoire of functions depending on their tissue location (NATHAN al. 1980; AUGER and ROSS 1993). They differ markedly in their response to pathogens, as described for *C. neoformans* (Levitz et al. 1997). Indeed, mouse resident peritoneal macrophages do not inhibit or kill *C. neoformans* if not treated with interferon γ. Human macrophages differ markedly from those of mice in their response to *C. neoformans*. Thus the fate of *B. anthracis* inside the macrophage may vary greatly, depending on the host species, anatomic location, and state of activation and differentiation. Image cytometry and expression technology with a high-sensitivity fluorescence-based reporter system (Zhang et al. 1991) have provided information about the molecular mechanisms associated with conversion of the germinated spore to a vegetative cell. Germination of *B. anthracis* within macrophages is closely followed by expression of the toxin genes (Guidi-Rontani et al. 1999a): genes encoding virulence factors such as the toxin transactivator AtxA, the lethal factor (LF), the protective antigen (PA), and the edema factor (EF) are rapidly expressed. The mature vegetative form has to escape from alveolar macrophage cells to multiply in the bloodstream with great rapidity. Encapsulated vegetative cells appear within 30 min after germination in vitro (Ezzell and Abshire 1995). It is not known whether capsulation starts within the macrophage, concomitant with toxin expression. Despite the work of Shafa and co-workers on intracellular multiplication (1966), it is still not clear whether *B. anthracis* multiplies within the macrophage. Indeed, these studies emphasize the importance of performing in vitro experiments under conditions that resemble, as closely as possible, those seen in vivo.

2.2 The Vegetative Form: An Extracellular Behavior

Analyses of blood cultures of infected rabbits (Bloom et al. 1947) and guinea pigs (Smith and Keppie 1954; Keppie et al. 1955) indicate that levels of bacteria in the blood rise steadily until the final hours of life, when they sharply increase to 10^7 (rabbits) and 10^9 (guinea pig) organisms or chains per milliliter of blood. Smith and Keppie (1954) demonstrated that death was dependent on bacteremia and that death was not a consequence of mechanical obstruction caused by such a high concentration of organisms. However, it must be noted that 15% of infected animals, for example, rabbits or monkeys, have fewer than 10^3 bacteria per milliliter of blood at the time of death (Bloom et al. 1947; Fritz et al. 1995). A point of commitment or point of no return has been identified: the fate of infected animals is determined when the number of bacteria present in the blood is two orders of magnitude lower than that at the time of death.

After challenge with fully virulent spores of the Vollum strain, polymorphonuclear leukocytes are recruited to the site of infection in the rat model (FISH et al. 1968). Mobilization of inflammatory cells has been suggested to be a major mechanism of host resistance (WELKOS et al. 1989), and chemotactic substances such as C5-derived chemoattractants may be important in the recruitment of macrophages (WELKOS et al. 1989). Vegetative forms survive as extracellular pathogens and, in contrast to spores, avoid phagocytosis by macrophages. Ingestion of the bacterium by host phagocytes is inhibited by the antiphagocytic poly-D-glutamic acid capsule because of its negative charge (TOMCSIK and SZONGOTT 1933; KEPPIE et al. 1963; STERNE 1937; EZZELL and WELKOS 1999), and *B. anthracis* isolates that lack the capsule are less virulent. In vitro *B. anthracis* has no capsule, but capsule synthesis is induced once it infects a host (PREISZ 1909): host signals, in particular a carbon dioxide concentration above 5%, activate the transcription of capsule and toxin genes (UCHIDA et al. 1997; SIRARD et al. 1994; KOEHLER et al. 1994).

3
Macrophage: A Target Cell for the Lethal Toxin

The molecular basis of microbial pathogenicity is usually complex and multifactorial. The harmful effects of numerous pathogenic bacteria are a consequence of the production of toxins; *B. anthracis* is one such bacterium. Since the characterization of anthrax toxins (SMITH and KEPPIE 1954; SMITH et al 1955), enormous effort has been devoted to the elucidation of the mechanism of their lethal effects.

As early as 1953, SMITH and co-workers suggested that the cause of death resulted from toxic factor(s) (SMITH et al. 1953, 1955; KEPPIE et al. 1953, 1955). In one experiment they demonstrated that sterile blood from infected guinea pigs caused physiopathological effects similar to these due to *B. anthracis* itself in uninfected guinea pigs (FRIEDLANDER 1986; LEPPLA 1995). The two *B. anthracis* toxins are in fact a tripartite system in which a common protein called the protective antigen (PA, 83 kDa), interacts separately with two other proteins, edema factor (EF, 89 kDa), which is a Ca^{2+}-calmodulin-dependent adenylate cyclase (LEPPLA 1982, 1984; LABRUYERE et al. 1990), and lethal factor (LF, 83 kDa), which is a metalloprotease. These toxins have biologically distinct effects (LEPPLA 1995).

Intravenous injection of LeTx (PA + LF) kills animals in a manner that closely mimics the natural systemic anthrax infection (Smith and Stanley 1962; Lincoln and Fish 1970; Leppla 1995). EdTx (PA + EF) causes profound edema when injected intradermally, a symptom observed in cases of cutaneous anthrax (Harris-Smith et al. 1958; Leppla 1982, 1995; Friedlander 1990). Lethal toxin-deficient strains are attenuated more than 1,000-fold, whereas inactivation of the EF gene reduces virulence only tenfold (Pezard et al. 1991; Brossier et al. 2000). Thus LF is essential for anthrax disease and lethality.

In 1986, Friedlander showed that the macrophage was the target cell of *B. anthracis* lethal toxin. In vitro, lethal toxin is cytolytic within 90–120 min for various primary macrophages isolated from mice, including C3H and the mouse macrophage-derived cell lines RAW264.7 and J774A.1. Although LeTx is internalized by other cell types, no other type of cultured cell appears to be affected (Friedlander 1986; Singh et al 1989; Friedlander et al. 1993a). LeTx triggers a cascade of physiological and biochemical alterations and then lysis of the macrophage (Hanna et al. 1992): (a) the earliest event, starting 45 min after challenge, is a large increase in the permeability of the plasma membrane to monovalent cations (^{22}Na and ^{86}Rb), causing ATP depletion; (b) by 60 min after challenge, this depletion of ATP induces an influx of Ca^{2+} (the membrane permeability to ^{45}Ca, ^{51}Cr, ^{36}Cl, $^{35}SO_4$, ^{3}H-amino acids and ^{3}H-uridine is altered) and lethal toxin-induced cytolysis is strictly dependent on this influx of Ca^{2+} (Bhatnagar et al. 1989); (c) at 75 min, the synthesis of macromolecules is inhibited and cellular lactate dehydrogenase leaks out of the cell; and (d) finally, at 90 min the macrophage lyses. Macrophages are therefore target cells for LeTx and appear to be a key element during toxemia (see also Sect. 5).

4
A Macrophage Molecular Target for LF

The cytotoxicity of LF is due to its zinc metalloprotease activity. LF contains a consensus zinc-binding site: $H^{686}EXXH^{690}$ (Klimpel et al. 1994) and is sensitive to protease inhibitors such as bestatin, chloromethyl ketones of leucine and phenylalanine. Indeed, these inhibitors prevent LeTx cytotoxicity (Menard et al. 1996). LF binds Zn^{2+} (Klimpel et al. 1994; Kochi et al. 1994) and substitution of the putative zinc binding histidines 686 or 690 by alanine reduced zinc binding. The mutant LeTx is only poorly cytotoxic to cultured cells and inactive on rats, and recombinant *B. anthracis* strains producing the mutated LF are devoid of lethality (KLIMPEL et al. 1994; BROSSIER et al. 2000). Thus LeTx is a zinc metalloprotease, but its physiological target remains unclear.

Recently, it was established that the mitogen-activated protein kinase kinases 1, 2, and 3 (MAPKK1, MAPKK2, and MAPKK3) are cleaved by LF within their N-termini both in vitro and in macrophage cytosol (DUESBERY et al. 1998; VITALE et al. 1998; PELLIZZARI et al. 1999). MAPKK is one of the three-kinase modules that compose the central core of each multienzyme mitogen-activated protein (MAP) kinase (MAPK) cascade. A phosphorylated and activated MAPKK kinase (MAPKKK) phosphorylates and activates a specific MAPKK, which then activates a specific MAPK (ANDERSON et al. 1990). The MAPK pathway relays environmental signals to the transcriptional machinery in the nucleus and thus modulates gene expression via a burst of protein phosphorylation (LEWIS et al. 1998). Inhibition of protein synthesis with cycloheximide fully inhibits LeTx cytotoxicity (BHATNAGAR and FRIEDLANDER 1994).

The large number of MAPKs could potentially allow differential phosphorylation of nuclear targets and thereby specific responses to upstream signals (YANG et al. 1998). LF cleaves MAPKK1 between amino acids 7 and 8 and MAPKK2 between residues 9 and 10, resulting in the loss of NH_2-terminal residues $PKKKPTP^7$ and $LARRKPVLP^9$, respectively (DUESBERY et al. 1998; VITALE et al. 1998). Consistent with this, LF cleaves in vitro synthetic peptides containing proline (HAMMOND and HANNA 1998), suggesting that proline residues constitute an important feature recognized by LF within the cleavage site. Using a molecular genetic method that screens for protein-protein interactions in yeast, VITALE and co-workers identified a cDNA for MAPKK2 that encodes an amino acid sequence lacking the cleavage site (residue 31 to residue 400). Consequently, we have to hypothesize that additional elements contribute to make this protein recognizable by LF. The amino acid sequences of the cleavage sites of MAPKK1 and 2 have only limited similarity with that of MAPKK3. It is therefore likely that specific tertiary structural elements make a large contribution to the target specificity of LF.

The cleavage of MAPKK1 and MAPKK2 by LF led to conflicting conclusions concerning the biological activities of the MAPKKs as modified by LF as well as to the outcome of such cleavages. DUESBERY and co-workers reported that LF prevented MAPKK1 and 2 from phosphorylating their substrates ERK1 and ERK2 in vitro (DUESBERY et al. 1998). The NH_2-terminal fragment of MAPKK1 and MAPKK2, containing MAPK binding site (FUKUDA et al. 1997) preceding the kinase domain, is lost after LF treatment, and thus LF may prevent the association of MAPKK1 with its substrate. In contrast, VITALE and co-workers showed that in vivo cleavage leads to phosphorylation of the MAPKK substrates ERK1 and ERK2 (VITALE et al. 1998). However, two lines of evidence suggest that proteolysis induced by LF does not result in loss of MAPKK activity: (a) a strict relationship between the onset of cell proliferation and the presence of the zinc metalloprotease-lethal toxin has been described (GUIDI-RONTANI et al. 1997); (b) MAPKK1 cleaved by LF may induce Golgi fragmentation during mitosis (COLANZI et al. 2000). Fragmentation of the Golgi stacks during mitosis is MAPKK1 dependent but does not require active ERK1 and ERK2. It appears that ERK1 and ERK2 are not the only MAPKK1 substrates.

Despite considerable insight into the structure-function relationship of LF and identification of putative cellular targets, the cytotoxicity mechanism of the lethal toxin remains unresolved. Note that macrophage cell lines and peritoneal macrophages isolated from mouse strains with different sensitivities to the cytocidal effects of LeTx give no evidence of a direct correlation between the LF-induced cleavage of MAPKKs and LF cytotoxicity (PELLIZZARI et al. 1999). The lack of correlation seems to indicate that other cytosolic targets of LF are responsible for the cytotoxicity. However, the differences between LF-sensitive and LF-resistant macrophages could be due to polymorphism in one or more components that act downstream from the cell signaling pathway, such as signaling molecule isoforms.

Recently, TANG and LEPPLA (1999) demonstrated that functional proteasome, a multicatalytic protease complex responsible for the degradation of ubiquitinated cellular proteins (WEISSMAN 1997), is essential for the cytotoxicity of LeTx. They suggest that LF cleaves an essential protein near the N terminus, as it does with MAPKKs, thereby converting it to a highly unstable protein and consequently making it a target for ubiquitination and proteasome degradation. Furthermore, ROBERTS and co-workers identified a single gene, on chromosome 11, designated *Ltx1*, that determines the susceptibility of mouse macrophages to LeTx (ROBERTS et al. 1998). Susceptibility was dominant to resistance, suggesting that resistance is caused by the absence of a molecule that acts downstream from the activity of LF.

The cytotoxicity of the lethal toxin is a complex phenomenon involving a multiplicity of substrates each belonging to complex and unsolved pathways. The MAPKK isoforms are key mediators of signal transduction from the cell surface to the nucleus (GOTOH and NISHIDA 1995). Seven different MAPKK have been identified (WU et al. 1997; FOLTZ et al. 1998) and compose three distinct MAPK cascades (ENGLISH et al 1999): (a) one cascade leads to the phospho-activation of the extracellular signal-regulated kinases (ERK1 and ERK2) with MAPKK1 and MAPKK2 as activators and MAPKK5 phospho-activating ERK5; (b) another cascade leads to the activation of the MAP kinase p38s via MAPKK3, MAPKK4 and MAPKK6; and (c) a third cascade leads to the activation of the c-jun N-terminal kinases (SAPK/JNK) via MAPKK4 and MAPKK7. Each MAPKK isoform tested (MAPKK1, MAPKK2 and MAPKK3) was cleaved by the lethal toxin. It would be interesting to test whether LF cleaves all MAPKK family members. LF recognizes and modifies several signaling molecule isoforms that have apparently redundant and interacting signal transfer functions (ENGLISH et al. 1999). In mammalian cells, MAPKKK such as MAPKKK1 can selectively activate two different MAPK pathways in response to different extracellular stimuli (YUJIRI et al. 1998). Moreover, nuclear substrates such as Elk-1 are substrates for three distinct classes of MAPKs (YANG et al. 1998). Possibly, the three distinct MAPK cascades interact, generating a complex network allowing fine regulation via the transmission of a signal. The mechanism may be dependent on the concentrations of the various signaling components (threshold stimuli required to trigger a response), their accessibility to each other (compartmentalization and/or simple diffusion), and the kinetics of the control of kinase activation. Note that it is difficult to identify mechanisms through which MAP-KK cleavage could lead to the rapid cell lysis observed in the presence of LeTx.

5 Contribution of Macrophage in Pathogenesis

The macrophage is a highly versatile cell type with an impressive repertoire of functions depending on location and activation status. The details of the contribution of macrophages as mediators of the symptoms and death due to systemic anthrax are unclear. Surprisingly, HANNA and coworkers showed that sublytic concentrations of lethal toxin, orders of magnitude lower than those required to induce lysis of RAW264.7 macrophages, induce these cells to express interleukin 1 (IL-1β) (DINARELLO 1991) and tumor necrosis factor (TNF-α) (VASSALI 1992) in vitro (HANNA et al. 1993). Interestingly, the signaling pathways involving MAPKK1, MAPKK2, and MAPKK3 are crucial in the activation of macrophages and are directly involved in the production of cytokines, i.e., in the biosynthesis of TNF-α, IL-1β, and IL-6 (LEE et al. 1994; BEYAERT et al. 1996). HANNA and co-workers reported the protection of mice from lethal toxin challenge by passive immunization against IL-1β and TNF-α or injection of an IL-1β receptor antagonist (HANNA et al. 1993). These results imply that systemic shock and death from anthrax may result primarily from the effects of high levels of proinflammatory cytokines, such as IL-1β and TNF-α, produced by macrophages after stimulation by the anthrax lethal toxin.

More recent studies have led to different conclusions about modulation of TNF-α and IL-1β production by lethal toxin (ERWIN et al. 2000). In contrast to the results of HANNA and co-workers, ERWIN and co-workers reported that LeTx does not induce the production of cytokines whether the LF subunit is present at lytic or at sublytic concentrations. Moreover, PELLIZZARI and co-workers and ERWIN and co-workers observed that LeTx inhibited the production of cytokines induced by LPS, suggesting that LF may suppress rather than induce cytokine production in macrophages (PELLIZZARI et al. 1999; ERWIN et al. 2000). These discrepancies concerning the molecular mechanism by which LeTx contributes to anthrax pathogenesis await clarification. HANNA and co-workers also reported that (a) mice specifically depleted of macrophages by silica (SiO_2) injections became resistant to the lethal toxin and (b) toxin sensitivity could be fully restored by coinjection of toxin-sensitive cultured macrophages, RAW264.7 cells. These experiments are in favor of a model whereby macrophages contribute to intoxication induced by the lethal toxin during infection (HANNA et al. 1993).

The edema toxin seems also to influence cytokine production, via enhancement of intracellular cAMP in human monocytes (HOOVER et al. 1994), by inducing IL-6 production. In contrast to this stimulatory effect on IL-6 production, EdTx induces little or no TNF-α production and strongly inhibits LPS-induced TNF-α. These regulatory phenomena were confirmed at the mRNA level. Interestingly, monocytes treated with dibutyryl cAMP, an active analog of cAMP, produce cytokines in a pattern identical to that of cells treated with edema toxin. EdTx inhibits the phagocytic activity of human polymorphonuclear neutrophils in vitro and blocks chemiluminescence induced in vitro by phorbol myristate acetate (PMA) (O'BRIEN et al. 1985). In contrast, EdTx stimulates chemotaxis of human polymorphonuclear neutrophils (WADE et al. 1985). Such stimulation may interfere with the normal modulation of chemotaxis by disrupting the chemoattractant gradient elicited during the infection. EdTx increases host susceptibility to infection by suppressing polymorphonuclear neutrophil function and thereby impairing host resistance.

B. anthracis diverts macrophage mechanisms involved in microbicidal activities and modulates the production of reactive oxygen and nitrogen intermediates (ROIs and RNIs, respectively). ROIs and RNIs are very reactive oxygen and nitrogen species and are toxic to the producing cell if they gain access to the cytosol (GALLIN and SNYDERMAN 1999). Their production must be restricted to subcellular compartment and tightly regulated to avoid overloading and then diffusion into cytosol, as this damages host tissues. Phagocytosis of apoptotic cells is one of the defense mechanisms against the damaging effects of released intracellular contents including superoxide anion, hydrogen peroxide, peroxynitrite, and hypochlorous acid (HENSON and JOHNSTON 1987). Modulation of the oxidative burst by lethal toxin has been described (HANNA et al. 1994): (a) RAW264.7 macrophage cells intoxicated with lethal toxin produce high concentrations of superoxide anion (220 nmol $O_2^-/10^7$ cells in 2 h) and stimulation of the oxidative burst is two to three times higher than that observed with potent activators of the NADPH oxidase complex such as PMA; (b) adding exogenous antioxidants, such as reducing agents (BME, DTT), organic solvents that trap free radicals (ethanol, DMSO), or oxygen scavenger (mepacrine), to macrophage cultures or boosting the endogenous macrophage glutathione antioxidant system significantly counteracts the cytotoxicity of the lethal toxin; and (c) macrophages completely deficient for ROI synthesis, for example, the murine line IC-21 and primary human monocytes from a patient with chronic granulomatous disease (CGD) (EZEKOWITZ 1992), are completely resistant to lethal toxin. These results strongly suggest that ROIs may regulate macrophage responses to lethal toxin.

Why the major ROI-producing cell, the neutrophil, is resistant to lethal toxin remains an intriguing question (WRIGHT and MANDELL 1986; O'BRIEN et al. 1985). The involvement of another macrophage-derived free radical gas, nitric oxide (NO), a mediator of the vascular and inflammatory response (HILL et al. 1996), should be investigated. Sublytic doses of LF reduce the release of NO induced by lipopolysaccharide/interferon γ (PELLIZZARI et al. 1999). Possibly, the reduction in the release of NO may contribute to the initial phase of infection by preventing microvascularization. As the release of NO is inhibited, the vessel cannot dilate, inhibiting the reduction of blood velocity. This would interfere with leukocyte recruitment at the site of acute inflammation.

The dysregulation of cytokine networks in macrophages may impair cellular antimicrobial responses and contribute to clinical signs and symptoms (Dixon et al. 1999). However, the relationships between the modulation of inflammatory mediators by LeTx, cytotoxicity, and pathogenicity need to be elucidated. Macrophages are guard cells, protecting against invading pathogens. Thus LeTx- and EdTx-mediated impairment of macrophage function is an effective strategy for pathogenicity. Inhibition of host inflammation and immune defenses creates advantageous conditions for the survival and multiplication of the invading bacteria.

6
Concluding Remarks

B. anthracis virulence is the sum of the contributions of factors involved in toxicity, growth, and persistence in the host. Numerous mechanisms involved in *B. anthracis* pathogenesis are centered on the macrophage. In the early steps of pathogenesis for the disease to be established, the spores must germinate in macrophages and emerge within an environment that allows rapid multiplication of capsulated vegetative forms in the animal body. An important goal for anthrax research is to identify the germinant specifically responsible for this germination within macrophage. During intoxication, the contribution of macrophage results from the subversion of various mechanisms of the host defense response against invading bacteria. The relationships between the intrinsic functions of macrophages and the response to *B. anthracis* are likely to be central to understanding *B. anthracis* pathogenesis. The complex network of such interactions is likely to become clearer thanks to identification of the entire repertoire of components from genome sequencing data. This may allow new therapeutic and preventative strategies to be developed.

Acknowledgements. We thank A. Moir and T. Read for generously providing *B. cereus* and *B. anthracis* sequence information and for stimulating discussions. We thank C. Montecucco for critical comments on this manuscript.

References

ABRAMOVA FA, GRINBERG LM, YAMPOLSKAYA OV, WALKER DH (1993) Pathology on inhalational anthrax in 42 cases from the Sverdlovsk outbreak of 1979. Proc Natl Acad Sci USA 90: 2291–2294

ANDERSON N, MALLER JL, TONKS N, STURGILL TW (1990) Requirement for integration of signals from two distinct phosphorylation pathways for activation of MAP kinase. Nature 343:651–653

ALPUCHE ARANDA CM, SWANSON JA, LOOMIS WP, MILLER SI (1993) *Salmonella typhimurium* activates virulence gene transcription within acidified macrophage phagosomes. Proc Natl Acad Sci USA 89:10079–10083

ARTHUR M, MOLINAS C, DEPARDIEU F, COURVALIN P (1993) Characterization of Tn1546, a Tn3-related transposon conferring glycopeptide resistance by synthesis of depsipeptide peptidoglycan precursors in *Enterococcus faecium* BM4147. J Bacteriol 175:117–127

AUGER MJ, ROSS JA (1993) The biology of the macrophage. In The Macrophage (Lewis CE and McGee JO, eds) Oxford, UK, Oxford University Press.

BARNES JM (1947) The development of anthrax following the administration of spores by inhalation. Brit J Exp Pathol XXVIII:385–394

BEALL FA, TAYLOR MJ, THORNE CB (1962) Rapid lethal effect in rats of a third component found upon fractionating the toxin of *Bacillus anthracis*. J Bacteriol 83:1274–1280

BEAMAN L, BEAMAN BL (1984) The role of oxygen and its derivatives in microbial pathogenesis and host defense. Annu Rev Microbiol 38:27–48

BEAMAN TC, PANKRATZ HS, GERHARDT P (1971) Paracrystalline sheets reaggregated from solubilised exosporium of *Bacillus cereus*. J Bacteriol 107:320–324

BECHTEL DB, BULLA LA (1976) Electron microscope study of sporulation and parasporal crystal formation in *Bacillus thuringiensis*. J Bacteriol 127:1472–1481

BERGER JA, MARR AG (1960) Sonic disruption of spores of *Bacillus cereus*. J Gen Microbiol 22:147–157

BEYAERT R, CUENDA A, VANDEN BERGHE W, PLAISANCE S, LEE JC, HAEGEMAN G, COHEN P, FIERS W (1996) The p38/RK mitogen-activated protein kinase pathway regulates interleukin-6 synthesis response to tumor necrosis factor. EMBO J 15: 1914–1923

BHATNAGAR R, FRIEDLANDER AM (1994) Protein synthesis is required for expression of anthrax lethal toxin cytotoxicity. Infect Immun 62:2958–2962

BHATNAGAR R, SINGH YS, LEPPLA SH, FRIEDLANDER AM (1989) Calcium is required for the expression of anthrax lethal toxin activity in the macrophage-like cell line J774A.1. Infect Immun 57:2107–2114

BINDER R, KRESS A, KAN G, HERRMANN K, KIRSCHFINK M (1999) Neutrophil priming by cytokines and vitamin D binding protein (Gc-globulin): impact on C5a-mediated chemotaxis, degranulation and respiratory burst. Mol Immunol 36: 885–892

BLOOM WL, MCGHEE WJ, CROMARTIE WJ, WATSON DWJ (1947) Studies on infection with *Bacillus anthracis*. J Infect Dis 80:137–142

BROSSIER F, WEBER-LEVY M, MOCK M, SIRARD JC (2000) Role of toxin functional domains in anthrax pathogenesis. Infect Immun 68:1781–1786

Buchner H, Merkel F, Enderlen E (1888) Untersuchungen über den Durchtritt von Infectionserregern durch die intacte Lungenoberfläche. Arch f Hyg 8:145–245

Caron E, Hall A (1998) Identification of two distinct mechanisms of phagocytosis controlled by different Rho GTPases. Science 282:1717–1721

Cataldi A, Labruyère E, Mock M (1990) Construction and characterization of a protective antigen-deficient *Bacillus anthracis* strain. Mol Microbiol 4: 1111–1117

Charlton S, Moir AJ, Baillie L, Moir A (1999) Characterization of the exosporium of *Bacillus cereus*. J Appl Microbiol 87:241–245

Clements MO, Moir A (1998) Role of the *gerI* operon of *Bacillus cereus* 569 in the response of spores to germinants. J Bacteriol 180: 6729–6735.

Cleveland EF, Gilvarg C (1975) Selective degradation of peptidoglycan from *Bacillus megaterium* spores during germination. In: Spores VI ed. Gerhardt P, Costilow RN, Sadoff HL, pp 458–464. Washington DC: American Society for Microbiology

Colanzi A, Deerinck TJ, Ellisman MH, Malhotra V (2000) A specific activation of the mitogen-activated protein kinase kinase 1 (MEK1) is required for golgi fragmentation during mitosis. J Cell Biol 149:331–339

Corfe BM, Sammons RL, Smith DA, Mauel C (1994) The *gerB* region of the *Bacillus subtilis* 168 chromosome encodes a homologue of the *gerA* spore germination operon. Microbiology 140: 471–478

Dalhammar G, Steiner H (1984) Characterization of inhibitor A, a protease from *Bacillus thuringiensis* which degrades attacins and cecropins, two classes of antibacterial proteins in insects. Eur J Biochem 139:247–252

Davaine C (1863) Recherches sur les infusoirs du sang dans la maladie connue sous le nom de "sang de rate". Comptes Rendus de l'Académie des Sciences LVII

Davies DG (1960) The influence of temperature and humidity on spore formation and germination in *Bacillus anthracis*. J Hyg Camb 58:177–186

De Bary A (1885) Vorlesungen über Bakter Verlag Wilhelm Engelmann, Leipzig

DesRosier JP, Lara JC (1984) Synthesis of the exosporium during sporulation of *Bacillus cereus*. J Gen Microbiol 130:935–940

De Vos V (1990) The ecology of anthrax in Kruger National Park, South Africa. Salisbury Med Bull Suppl 68:19–23

Dinarello CA (1991) Interleukin-1 and interleukin-1 antagonism. Blood 77:1627–1652

Dixon TC, Meselson M, Guillemin J, Hanna PC (1999) Anthrax. N Engl J Med 9:815–826

Duesbery NS, Vande Woude GF (1999) Anthrax toxins. Cell Mol Life Sci 55:1599–1609

Duesbery NS, Webb CP, Leppla SH, Gordon VM, Klimpel KR, Copeland TD, Ahn NG, Oskarsson MK, Fukasawa K, Paull KD, Vandewoude GF (1998) Proteolytic inactivation of MAP-kinase-kinase by anthrax lethal factor. Science 280:734–737

Eissenberg GL, Goldman WE, Schlesinger PH (1993) *Histoplasma capsulatum* modulates the acidification of phagolysosomes. J Exp Med 177:1605–1611

Enderlen E (1889) Ueber den Durchtritt von Milzbrandsporen durch die intacte Lungenoberfläche des Schafes. Deutsche Z f Thiermedicin u Vergeich Path 15:50–56

English J, Pearson G, Wilsbacher J, Swantek J, Karandikar M, Xu S, Cobb MH (1999) New insights into the control of MAP kinase pathways. Exp Cell Res 25: 255–270

ERRINGTON J (1993) *Bacillus subtilis* sporulation: regulation of gene expression and control of morphogenesis. Microbiol Rev 57: 1–33

ERWIN JL, LITTLE SF, FRIEDLANDER AM, DASILVA L, BAVARI S, CHANH TC (2000) Macrophage-derived cell lines do not express pro-inflammatory cytokines after exposure to anthrax lethal toxin. American Society for Microbiology Abstract #E-79

EZEKOWITZ RAB (1992) Chronic granulomatous disease: an update and a paradigm for the use of interferon-gamma as adjunct immunotherapy in infectious diseases. Current Top Microbiol Immunol 181:283–292

EZZELL JW, ABSHIRE TG (1995) Encapsulation of *Bacillus anthracis* spores and spore identification. Salisbury Medical Bulletin. Proceedings of the International Workshop on Anthrax. Winchester, England, Sept. 19–21

EZZELL JW, WELKOS SL (1999) The capsule of *Bacillus anthracis*, a review. J Appl Microbiol 87:250–257

FEAVERS IM, FOULKES J, SETLOW B, SUN D, NICHOLSON W, SELOW P, MOIR A (1990) The regulation of transcription of the *gerA* spore germination operon of *Bacillus subtilis*. Mol Microbiol 4:275–282

FISH DC, KLEIN F, LINCOLN RE, WALKER JS, DOBBS JP (1968) Pathophysiological changes in the rat associated with anthrax toxin. J Infect Dis 118:114–124

FLÜGGE C (1886) Die mikroorganismen. Verlag FCW Vogel, Leipzig S: 607–608

FOLTZ IN, GERL RE, WIELER JS, LUCKACH M, SALMON RA, SCHRADER JW (1998) Human mitogen-activated protein kinase kinase 7 (MKK7) is a highly conserved c-jun N-terminal kinase/stress-activated protein kinase (JNK/SAPK) activated by environmental stresses and physiological stimuli. J Biol Chem 273:9344–9351

FOSTER SJ (1994) The role and regulation of cell wall structural dynamics during differentiation of endospore-forming bacteria. J Appl Bacteriol Symp Suppl 76:25S–39S

FOSTER SJ, JOHNSTONE K (1990) Pulling the trigger: the mechanism of bacterial spore germination. Mol Microbiol 4:137–141.

FRIEDLANDER AM (1986) Macrophages are sensitive to anthrax lethal toxin through an acid-dependent process. J Biol Chem 261:7123–7126

FRIEDLANDER AM (1990) The anthrax toxin. In: Saelinger CB (ed) Trafficking of bacterial toxins. CRC Press, Boca Raton, Florida

FRIEDLANDER AM, BHATNAGAR R, LEPPLA SH, JOHNSON L, SINGH Y (1993a) Characterization of macrophage sensitivity and resistance to anthrax lethal toxin. Infect Immun 61:245–252

FRIEDLANDER AM, WELKOS SL, PITT MLM, EZZELL JW, WORSHAM PL, ROSE KJ (1993b) Postexposure prophylaxis against experimental inhalation anthrax. J Infect Dis 167:1239–1242

FRITZ DL, JAAX NK, LAWRENCE WB, DAVIS KJ, PITT MLM, EZZELL JW, FRIEDLENDER AM (1995) Pathology of experimental inhalation anthrax in the Rhesus monkey. Lab Invest 73:691–702

FUKUDA M, GOTOH Y, NISHIDA E (1997) Interaction of MAP kinase with MAP kinase kinase: its possible role in the control of nucleocytoplasmic transport of MAP kinase. EMBO J 16:1901–1908

GALLIN JI, SNYDERMAN R (1999) Inflammation. Basic principles and clinical correlates. Raven Press, New York

Garcia-Patrone M, Tandercarz JS (1995) A glycoprotein multimer from *Bacillus thuringiensis* sporangia: Dissociation into subunits and sugar composition. Mol Cell Biochem 145:29–37

Gerhardt P (1967) Cytology of *Bacillus anthracis*. Fed Proc 26:1504–1517

Gerhardt P, Ribi E (1964) Ultrastructure of the exosporium enveloping spores of *Bacillus cereus*. J Bact 88:1774–1789

Gleiser CA, Berdjis CC, Hartman HA, Gochenour WS (1963) Pathology of experimental respiratory anthrax in Macaca mulatta. Brit J Exp Pathol 44:416–426

Gotoh Y, Nishida E (1995) The MAP kinase cascade: Its role in Xenopus oocytes, eggs and embryos. In: Meijer L, Guidet S, Tung HYL (eds) Progress in cell cycle research. Plenum Press, New York

Gould GW (1977) Recent advances in the understanding of resistance and dormancy in bacterial spores. J Appl Bacteriol 42:297–309

Green BD, Battisti L, Koehler TM, Thorne CB, Ivins BE (1985) Demonstration of a capsule plasmid in *Bacillus anthracis*. Infect Immun 49: 291–297

Greenberg S (1999) Modular components of phagocytosis. Leukoc Biol 66:712–177

Greenberg S, El Khoury J, Di Virgilio F, Kaplan EM, Silverstein SC (1991) Ca^{++}-independent F-actin assembly and disassembly during Fc receptor-mediated phagocytosis in mouse macrophages. J Cell Biol 113:757–767

Guidi-Rontani C, Duflot E, Mock M (1997) Anthrax lethal toxin-induced mitogenic response of human T-cells FEMS Microbiol Lett 157:285–289

Guidi-Rontani C, Pereira Y, Ruffie S, Sirard JC, Mock M (1999b) Identification and characterization of a germination operon on the virulence plasmid pXO1 of *Bacillus anthracis*. Mol Microbiol 33:407–414

Guidi-Rontani C, Weber-Levy M, Labruyere E, Mock M (1999a) Germination of *Bacillus anthracis* spores within alveolar macrophages. Mol Microbiol 31:9–17

Hachisuka Y (1969) Germination of *B. anthracis* spores in the peritoneal cavity of rats and establishment of anthrax. Jpn J Microbiol 13:199–207

Hachisuka Y, Kojima K, Sato T (1966) Fine filaments on the outside of the exosporium of *Bacillus anthracis* spores. J Bact 91:2382–2384

Hackstadt T (1983) Estimation of the cytoplasmic pH of *Coxiella burnetii* and effect of substrate oxidation on proton motive force. J Bact 154: 591–597

Halvorson HO (1997) Two generations of spore research: from father to son. Microbiologia SEM 13:131–148

Hammond SE, Hanna PC (1998) Lethal factor active-site mutations affect catalytic activity in vitro. Infect Immun 66:2374–2378

Hampton MB, Kettle AJ, Winterbourn CC (1998) Inside the neutrophil phagosome: oxidants, myeloperoxidase, and bacterial killing. Blood 92:3007–3017

Hanna PC, Acosta D, Collier RJ (1993) On the role of macrophages in anthrax. Proc Natl Acad Sci USA 90:10198–10201

Hanna PC, Kochi S, Collier RJ (1992) Biochemical and physiological changes induced by anthrax lethal toxin in J774 macrophage-like cells. Molec Biol of the cell 1:7–18

Hanna PC, Kruskal BA, Ezekowitz RAB, Bloom BR, Collier RJ (1994) Role of macrophage oxidative burst in the action of anthrax lethal toxin. Mol Med 1:7–18

Harris-Smith PW, Smith H, Keppie J (1958) Production in vitro of the toxin of *Bacillus anthracis* previously recognized in vivo. J Gen Microbiol 19: 91–103

Henson PM, Johnston RB Jr (1987) Tissue injury in inflammation. Oxidants, proteinases, and cationic proteins. J Clin Invest 79:669–674

Hill JR, Corbett JA, Kwon G, Marshall CA, McDaniel ML (1996) Nitric oxide regulates interleukin 1 bioactivity released from murine macrophages. J Biol Chem 271:22672–22678

Hills GM (1949) Chemical factors in the germination of spore-bearing aerobes. The effects of amino-acids on the germination of *Bacillus anthracis*, with some observations on the relation of optical form to biological activity. Biochem J 45: 363–370

Hoffmaster AR, Koehler TM (1999) Autogenous regulation of the *Bacillus anthracis pag* operon. J Bacteriol 181:4485–4492

Hoover DL, Friedlander AM, Rogers LC, Yoon IK, Warren RL, Cross AS (1994) Anthrax edema toxin differentially regulates lipopolysaccharide-induced monocyte production of tumor necrosis factor alpha and interleukin-6 by increasing intracellular cyclic AMP. Infect Immun 62:4432–4439

Inglesby TV (1999) Anthrax: A possible case history. Emerg Infect Dis 5:556–560

Irie R, Fujita YY, Kobayashi M (1996) Nucleotide sequence and gene organization of the *gerK* spore germination locus of *Bacillus subtilis* 168. J Gen Appl Microbiol 42: 141–153

Keppie J, Harris-Smith PW, Smith H (1963) The chemical basis of the virulence of *Bacillus anthracis.* IX: Its aggressins and their mode of action. Brit J Exp Pathol 44: 446–453

Keppie J, Smith H, Harris-Smith PW (1953) The chemical basis of the virulence of *Bacillus anthracis.* II: some biological properties of bacterial products. Brit J Exp Pathol 37: 446–453

Keppie J, Smith H, Harris-Smith PW (1955) The chemical basis of the virulence of *Bacillus anthracis.* III: The role of the terminal bacteraemia in death of guinea-pigs from anthrax. Brit J Exp Pathol 36: 315–322

Kerr JR (1999) Cell adhesion molecules in the pathogenesis of and host defence against microbial infection. Mol Pathol 52:220–230

Klein F, Walker JS, Fitzpatrick DF, Lincoln RE, Mahlandt BG, Jones WI et al. (1966) Pathophysiology of anthrax. J Infect Dis 116:123–138

Klimpel KR, Arora N, Leppla SH (1994) Anthrax toxin lethal factor contains a zinc metalloprotease consensus sequence which is required for lethal toxin activity. Mol Microbiol 13:1093–1100

Koch R (1876) Die etiologie der milzbrand krankheit hegrundet auf die entwickelungsgeschichte des *Bacillus anthracis.* Beitr Biol Pflanz 2:277–283

Kochi SK, Schiavo G, Mock M, Montecucco C (1994) Zinc content of the *Bacillus anthracis* lethal factor. FEMS Microbiol Lett 124:343–348

Koehler TM, Dai Z, Kaufman-Yarbray M (1994) Regulation of the *Bacillus anthracis* protective antigen gene: CO_2 and a *trans*-acting element activate transcription from one of two promoters. J Bacteriol 176: 586–595.

Labruyere E, Mock M, Ladant D, Michelson S, Gilles AM, Laoide B, Barzu O (1990) Characterization of ATP and calmodulin-binding properties of a truncated form of *Bacillus anthracis* adenylate cyclase Biochemistry 29:4922–4928

Laforce FM, Bumford FH, Feeley JC, Stokes SL, Snow DB (1969) Epidemiologic study of a fatal case of inhalation anthrax. Arch Environ Health 18: 798–805

Lee JC, Laydon JT, McDonnell PC, Gallagher TF, Kumar S, Green D, McNulty D, Blumenthal MJ Heys JR, Landvatter SW, et al. (1994) A protein kinase involved in the regulation of inflammatory cytokine biosynthesis. Nature 372: 739–746

Leppla SH (1982) Anthrax toxin edema factor: a bacterial adenylate cyclase that increases cyclic AMP concentrations of eukaryotic cells. Proc Natl Acad Sci USA 79:3162–3166

Leppla SH (1984) *Bacillus anthracis* calmodulin-dependent adenylate cyclase: chemical and enzymatic properties and interactions with eukaryotic cells. In: Greengard P, Robison BA (eds) Advances in cyclic nucleotide and protein phosphorylation research. Raven Press, New York, pp 189–198

Leppla SH (1991) The anthrax toxin complex. In: Alouf JE, Freer JH (eds) Sourcebook of bacterial protein toxins. Academic, London, pp 277–301

Leppla SH (1995) Anthrax toxins. In: Moss J, Iglewski B, Vaughan M, Tu AT (eds) Bacterial toxins and virulence factors in disease. Dekker, New York, pp 543–572

Levitz SM, Harrison TS, Tabuni A, Liu X (1997) Chloroquine induces human mononuclear phagocytes to inhibit and kill *Cryptococcus neoformans* by a mechanism independent of iron deprivation. J Clin Invest 100:1640–1646

Lewis TS, Shapiro PS, Ahn NG (1998) Signal transduction through MAP kinase cascades. Adv Cancer Res 74:49–139

Lincoln RE, Fish DC (1970) Anthrax toxin. In: Montie TC, Kadis S, Ajl SJ (eds) Microbial toxins, vol III. Academic Press, New York, pp 361–414

Lincoln RE, Hodges DR, Klein F, Mahlandt BG, Jones WI, Haines BW, Rhian MA, Walker JS (1965) Role of the lymphatics in the pathogenesis of anthrax. J Infect Dis 115:481–94

Manchee RJ, Broster MG, Melling J, Henstridge RM, Stagg ZJ (1981) *Bacillus anthracis* on Gruinard Island. Nature 294: 254–255

Manchee RJ, Broster MG, Stagg AJ, Hibbs SE, Patience B (1990) Out of Gruinard Island, No. 68 Special Supplement, pp 17–18. In: Turnbull PCB (ed), Proceedings of the International Workshop on "Anthrax", Winchester, England, April 11–13, 1989. Salisbury Medical Bulletin.

Matz LL, Beaman TC, Gerhardt P (1970) Chemical composition of exosporium from spores of *Bacillus cereus*. J Bacteriol 101:196–201

McCann KP, Robinson C, Sammons RL, Smith DA, Corfe BM (1996) Alanine germination receptors of *Bacillus subtilis*. Lett Appl Microbiol 23:290–294

Metchnikoff E (1905) Immunity in infective diseases. Cambridge University Press, London

Miles J, Latter PM, Smith IR, Heal OW (1988) Ecological aspects of killing *Bacillus anthracis* on Gruinard Island with formaldehyde. Reclamation Revegetation Res 6:271–283

Moir A, Kemp EH, Robinson C, Corfe BM (1994) The genetic analysis of bacterial spore germination. J Appl Bact 76:9S-16 S

Moir A, Smith DA (1990) The genetics of bacterial spore germination. Annu Rev Microbiol 44:531–553

Menard A, Papini E, Mock M, Montecucco C (1996) The cytotoxic activity of *Bacillus anthracis* lethal factor is inhibited by leukotriene A4 hydrolase and metallopeptidase inhibitors. Biochem J 320:687–691

MOULDER JW (1985) Comparative biology of intracellular parasitism. Microbiol Rev 49:298–337

MURRELL WG (1969) Chemical composition of spores and spore structures. In: Gould GW, Hurst A (eds), The bacterial spore. Academic Press, London, New York. pp 215–273

NATHAN CF, MURRAY HW, COHN ZA (1980) The macrophage as an effector cell. N Engl J Med 303:622–626

O'BRIEN J, FRIEDLANDER AM, DREIER T, EZZELL J, LEPPLA SH (1985) Effect of anthrax toxin components on human neutrophils. Infect Immun 46:306–310

OHYE DF, MURRELL WG (1973) Exosporium and spore coatformation in *Bacillus cereus* T. J Bacteriol 115:1179–1190

OKINAKA RT, CLOUD K, HAMPTON O, HOFFMASTER AR, HILL KK, KEIM P, KOEHLER TM, LAMKE G, KUMANO S, MAHILLON J, MANTER D, MARTINEZ Y, RICKE D, SVENSSON R, JACKSON PJ (1999) Sequence and organization of pXO1, the large *Bacillus anthracis* plasmid harboring the anthrax toxin genes. J Bacteriol 181:6509–6515

PASTEUR (1877) Etude sur la maladie du charbonneuse. Comptes Rendus de l'Académie des Sciences LXXXIV:900–906

PELLIZZARI R, GUIDI-RONTANI C, VITALE G, MOCK M, MONTECUCCO C (1999) Anthrax lethal factor cleaves MKK3 in macrophages and inhibits the LPS/IFN-induced release of NO and TNF. FEBS Lett 462:199–204

PEZARD C, BERCHE P, MOCK M (1991) Contribution of individual toxin components to the virulence of *Bacillus anthracis*. Infect Immun 59:3472–3477

PREISZ H (1909) Experimentelle Studien über Virulenz, Empfänglichkeit und Immunität beim Milzbrand. Zeitschr Immunitätsf 5: 341–452

ROBERTS JE, WATTERS JW, BALLARD JD, DIETRICH WF (1998) Ltx1, a mouse locus that influences the susceptibility of macrophages to cytolysis caused by intoxication with *Bacillus anthracis* lethal factor, maps to chromosome 11. Mol Microbiol 29: 581–591

ROSS JM (1957) The pathogenesis of anthrax following the administration of spores by the respiratory route. J Path Bact LXXIII:485–494

RUSSELL AD (1990) Bacterial spores and chemical sporicidal agents. Clin Microbiol Rev 3:99–119

SAKAE Y, YASUDA Y, TOCHIKUBO K (1995) Immunoelectron microscopic localization of one of the spore germination proteins, GerAB, in *Bacillus subtilis* spores. J Bacteriol 177:6294–6296

SHAFA F, MOBERLY BJ, GERHARDT P (1966) Cytological features of anthrax spores phagocytized in vitro by rabbit alveolar macrophages. J Infect Dis 116:401–413

SINGH Y, LEPPLA SH, BHATNAGAR R, FRIEDLANDER AM (1989) Internalization and processing of *Bacillus anthracis* lethal toxin by toxin-sensitive and -resistant cells. J Biol Chem 264:11099–11102

SIRARD JC, MOCK M, FOUET A (1994) The three *Bacillus anthracis* toxin genes are coordinately regulated by carbonate and temperature. J Bact 176:5188–5192

SMITH H., KEPPIE J (1954) Observations on experimental anthrax: Demonstration of a specific lethal factor produced in vivo by *Bacillus anthracis*. Nature 173:869–870

SMITH H, KEPPIE J, STANLEY JL (1953) The chemical basis of the virulence of *Bacillus anthracis*. I: properties of bacteria grown in vivo and preparation of extracts. Brit J Exp Pathol 34:477–485

Smith H, Keppie J, Stanley JL (1955) The chemical basis of the virulence of *Bacillus anthracis*. V: The specific toxin produced by *B. anthracis* in vivo. Brit J Exp Pathol 36:460–472

Smith H, Stanley JL (1962) The terminal phase of anthrax. Brit J Exp Pathol 43: 684–686

Stephen J (1981) Anthrax toxin. In: Dorner F, Drews J (eds) Anthrax toxin. Pergamon Press, Oxford, pp 501–513

Stephen J (1986) Anthrax toxin. In: Dorner F, Drews J (eds) Pharmacology of bacterial toxins. Pergamon, Oxford, pp 381–395

Sterne M (1937) Variation in *Bacillus anthracis*. Onderstepoort J Vet Sci Anim Ind 8: 271–349

Tang G, Leppla SH (1999) Proteasome activity is required for anthrax lethal toxin to kill macrophages. Infect Immun 67:3055–3060

Thompson HA, Williams JC (1991) in Q fever: The biology of *Coxiella burnetti*. J.C. Williams, H.A. Thompson, Eds. (CRC Press, Boston) 117–129.

Titball RW, Manchee RJ (1987) Factors affecting the germination of spores of *Bacillus anthracis*. J Applied Bact 62:269–273

Tomcsik J, Bouille M, Baumann-Grace JB (1959) Réaction spécifique de l'exosporium chez *Bacillus cereus* et *Bacillus anthracis*. Schweiz Z Path Bakt 22:630-640

Tomcsik J, Szongott H (1933) Ueber ein spezifisches protein der kaspel des milzbrandbazillus. Zeitschr Immunitätsf 78:86–99

Uchida I, Hornung JM, Thorne CB, Klimpel KR, Leppla SH (1993) Cloning and characterization of a gene whose product is a trans-activator of anthrax toxin synthesis. J Bacteriol 175: 5329–5338

Uchida I, Makino S, Sekizaki T, Terakado N (1997) Cross-talk to the genes for *Bacillus anthracis* capsule synthesis by atxA, the gene encoding the trans-activator of anthrax toxin synthesis. Mol Microbiol 23:1229–1240

Vassali P (1992) The pathophysiology of tumor necrosis factor. Annu Rev Immunol 10:411–452

Vitale G, Pellizzari R, Recchi C, Napolitani G, Mock M, Montecucco C (1998) Anthrax lethal factor cleaves the N-terminus of MAPKKs and induces tyrosine/threonine phosphorylation of MAPKs in cultured macrophages. Biochem Biophys Res Commun 248:706–711

Wade BH, Wright GG, Hewlett EL, Leppla SH, Mandell GL (1985) Anthrax toxin components stimulate chemotaxis of human polymorphonuclear neutrophils. Proc Soc Exp Biol Med 179:159–162

Weissman AM (1997) Regulating protein degradation by ubiquitination. Immunol Today 18:189–98

Welhrli E, Scherrer P, Kübler O (1980) The crystalline layers in spores of *Bacillus cereus* and *Bacillus thuringiensis* studied by freeze-etching and high resolution electron microscopy. Eur J Cell Biol 20:283–289

Welkos SL, Trotter RW, Friedlander AM (1989) Resistance to the Sterne strain of *B. anthracis*: phagocytic cell responses of resistant and susceptible mice. Microbial Pathogenesis 7:15–35

Wright GG, Mandell GL (1986) Anthrax toxin blocks priming of neutrophils by lipopolysaccharide and by muramyl dipeptide. J Exp Med 164:1700–1709

Wu Z, Wu J, Jacinto E, Karin M (1997) Molecular cloning and characterization of human JNKK2, a novel jun NH(2)-terminal kinase-specific kinase. Molec Cell Biol 17:7407–7416

Yasuda Y, Tochikubo K (1984) Effect of glucose on the interaction of hydrophobic compounds with the alanine receptor field of *Bacillus subtilis* spores during initiation of germination. Microbiol Immunol 28:1203–1210

Yasuda Y, Sakae Y, Tochikubo K (1996) Immunological detection of the GerA spore germination proteins in the spore integuments of *Bacillus subtilis* using scanning electron microscopy. FEMS Microbiol Lett 139:235–238

Yang SH, Whitmarsh AJ, Davis RJ, Sharrocks AD (1998) Differential targeting of MAP kinases to the ETS-domain transcription factor Elk-1. EMBO J 17:1740–1749

Yujiri T, Sather S, Fanger GR, Johnson GL (1998) Role of MEKK1 in cell survival and activation of JNK and ERK pathways defined by targeted gene disruption. Science 282:1911–1914

Zaucha GM, Pitt MLM, Estep J, Ivins BE, Friedlander AM (1998) The pathology of experimental anthrax in rabbits exposed by inhalation and subcutaneous inoculation. Arch Pathol Lab Med 122:982–992

Zhang YZ, Naleway JJ, Larison KD, Huang Z, Haugland RP (1991) Detecting lacZ gene expression in living cells with new lipophilic, fluorogenic beta-galactosidase substrates. FASEB J 5: 3108–3113

Zuberi AR, Feavers IM, Moir A (1985) Identification of three complementation units in the *gerA* spore germination locus of *B. subtilis* 168. J Bacteriol 162: 756–762

Zuberi AR, Moir A, Feavers IM (1987) The nucleotide sequence and gene organization of the gerA spore germination operon of *Bacillus subtilis* 168. Gene 51:1–11

CHAPTER 7

Bacillus anthracis Genetics and Virulence Gene Regulation

T. M. KOEHLER

Abstract. The *Bacillus anthracis* genome consists of an approximately 5.3-Mb chromosome and two plasmids, pXO1 (182 kb) and pXO2 (96 kb). Genetic analysis has focused primarily on the structural genes for the anthrax toxin proteins, *pagA*, *lef*, and *cya*, the biosynthetic genes for capsule synthesis, *capB*, *capC*, and *capA*, and a gene associated with depolymerization of capsule, *dep*. The three toxin genes are located at distinct loci on pXO1, while the *cap* and *dep* genes are arranged in an apparent

T. M. KOEHLER
Department of Microbiology and Molecular Genetics, University of Texas Medical School, Houston, TX 77030, USA, Email: tkoehler@utmmg.med.uth.tmc.edu.

operon on pXO2. Additional genes that may play a role in *B. anthracis* virulence include the germination operon *gerX* and the general stress transcription factor *sigB*. Host-related signals affecting transcription of the toxin and capsule genes include temperature (37 °C) and bicarbonate/CO_2. The *B. anthracis* plasmids carry two regulatory genes that share little sequence similarity with regulators in other bacteria. The pXO1-encoded gene *atxA* positively controls expression of the toxin and capsule genes, and has been implicated in control of other genes of unknown function. *atxA* mutants are avirulent in mice, and mice infected with *atxA*-null strains show a decreased immunological response to the toxin proteins. The pXO2-encoded regulator, *acpA*, shares sequence similarity with *atxA*. Yet *acpA* function appears to be restricted to positive control of capsule gene expression. The chromosomal gene *abrB*, a homologue of a well-characterized *B. subtilis* transition state regulator, controls growth phase-specific transcription of the toxin genes. Genetic manipulation of *B. anthracis* can be achieved by using natural means of DNA transfer and by electroporation of recombinant DNAs into *B. anthracis*. Genetic exchange can occur between *B. anthracis* strains and between *B. anthracis* and closely-related species. Although pXO1 and pXO2 are not self-transmissible, these plasmids and others can be transferred by conjugative plasmids originating in *B. thuringiensis*. Generalized transducing phage that permit inter-species transfer of chromosomal and plasmid DNA have also been described.

1 Introduction

Historically, the most fundamental discovery regarding the genetic composition of *B. anthracis* was the detection of two large resident plasmids, pXO1 (originally known as pBA1) and pXO2 (previously also known as pTE702). The discovery of these plasmids revealed the first clues regarding the genetic basis for toxin and capsule synthesis and insight regarding Pasteur's live attenuated anthrax vaccines (see chapter 3 of this volume). It also spurred the development of methods to transfer genetic material into and out of *B. anthracis* and set the stage for cloning of the toxin and capsule genes and monitoring their expression.

In the early 1980s improved methods for isolation of extrachromosomal DNA in bacteria revealed the presence of two different plasmids in *B. anthracis*. When the plasmid content of fully virulent and attenuated strains was compared, synthesis of the anthrax toxin proteins was associated with pXO1 and capsule biosynthesis was associated with pXO2. Proof of the relationship between plasmid content and the toxin and capsule phenotypes was obtained when strains were cured of pXO1 and pXO2 and the resulting phenotypes were examined. Loss of pXO1, resulting from growth of *B. anthracis* at 42 °C or in the presence of chemical agents, rendered strains unable to produce the three toxin proteins (MIKESELL et al. 1983). Loss of pXO2 after growth in sublethal concentrations of novobiocin resulted in noncapsulated strains (GREEN et al. 1985; UCHIDA et al. 1985). When the plasmids were reintroduced into cured isolates, toxin and capsule synthesis were restored (GREEN et al. 1985, 1989).

Once the associations of toxin synthesis with pXO1 and capsule synthesis with pXO2 were established, the structural genes for the toxin proteins *pagA* (originally named *pag*), encoding protective antigen (PA); *cya*, encoding edema factor (EF); and *lef*, encoding lethal factor (LF), were cloned, sequenced, and mapped to a restriction enzyme cleavage map of pXO1 (VODKIN and LEPPLA 1983; WELKOS et al. 1988; TIPPETTS and ROBERTSON 1988; ROBERTSON et al. 1988; MOCK et al. 1988; BRAGG and ROBERTSON 1989; ROBERTSON et al. 1990). The genes required for biosynthesis of the capsule, *capB*, *capC*, *capA*, and a gene associated with capsule depolymerization, *dep*, were cloned, sequenced, and mapped to pXO2 (UCHIDA et al. 1993b, 1987; MAKINO et al. 1988, 1989).

The complete DNA sequences of pXO1 and pXO2 are now known (AF065404 and AF188935), and sequence annotation suggests that approximately 65 % of the plasmid DNA represents coding regions (OKINAKA et al. 1999). Together, pXO1 and pXO2 may encode as many as 200 proteins, yet little is known about the expression or function of these potential genes (see chapter 2 of this volume). The only phenotype associated with pXO2 is the ability to synthesize capsule. In addition to the capsule biosynthetic and depolymerization genes, pXO2 harbors a *trans*-acting regulator of capsule gene expression called *acpA* (see below). No other pXO2-encoded genes have been characterized. Unlike pXO2, pXO1 is associated with a number of phenotypes. In addition to the inability to synthesize toxin, $pXO1^-$ strains grow more poorly on certain minimal media, are more sensitive to some bacteriophages, produce less capsule material, and sporulate earlier and at a higher frequency than $pXO1^+$ strains (THORNE 1993). Some of these phenotypes are associated with the pXO1-encoded regulatory gene, *atxA* (see below). Other pXO1 genes that have been characterized include: (1) *pagR*, a gene that is cotranscribed with *pagA* and acts as a weak repressor of the *pagAR* operon (HOFFMASTER and KOEHLER 1999); (2) *gerXB*, *gerXA*, and *gerXC*, genes of an operon that affect germination in vivo and in vitro within phagocytic cells (GUIDI-RONTANI et al. 1999a); and (3) *topX*, a type 1 topoisomerase gene that may be involved in plasmid stability (FOUET et al. 1994).

2 Host-Related Cues and Virulence Gene Expression

In terms of gene regulation, the most thoroughly studied *B. anthracis* genes are the structural genes for the three anthrax toxin proteins and the genes required for biosynthesis of the *B. anthracis* capsule. Early investigations of toxin and capsule synthesis by *B. anthracis* growing in batch culture indicated that synthesis of these essential virulence factors is enhanced when *B. anthracis* is grown in defined media containing bicarbonate or dissolved CO_2. CO_2/bicarbonate-enhanced toxin and capsule gene expression is at the level of transcription (BARTKUS and LEPPLA 1989; CATALDI et al. 1992; KOEHLER et al. 1994; SIRARD et al. 1994; UCHIDA et al. 1997; VIETRI et al. 1995). Toxin gene promoter activity and toxin proteins yields are highest at late log phase when grown in CA or R medium containing bicarbonate or in an elevated (5% or greater) CO_2 atmosphere (KOEHLER et al. 1994; LEPPLA 1988; LEPPLA 1991; SIRARD et al. 1994). At late log phase in batch culture, expression of a *pag-lacZ* transcriptional fusion on pXO1 is induced five- to eightfold during growth in 5% CO_2 compared with growth in air (0.03% CO_2) (KOEHLER et al. 1994). Activity of a *capB-lacZ* transcriptional fusion on pXO2 is induced approximately 25-fold during growth in medium containing bicarbonate (GUIGNOT et al. 1997). The response to CO_2/bicarbonate is specific and not simply due to the buffering capacity of dissolved bicarbonate during bacterial growth or to decreased oxygen levels (THORNE 1993).

In addition to bicarbonate, temperature has been shown to affect toxin synthesis. Transcription of the toxin genes is elevated when cells are cultured at 37 °C relative to lower temperatures. When cells are grown in elevated CO_2, promoter activity of the three toxin genes is increased four- to sixfold during incubation at 37 °C compared with incubation at 28 °C (SIRARD et al. 1994). No temperature effects on capsule gene expression have been reported.

3
Transcriptional Analysis of the Toxin and Capsule Genes

The three structural genes for the toxin proteins are located noncontiguously on a 46.6-kb pathogenicity island of pXO1 (OKINAKA et al. 1999). Results of Northern hybridization experiments indicate that the *cya* and *lef* genes are expressed as monocistronic transcripts (T. Koehler, unpublished data). The *cya* gene has one apparent transcriptional start site, located 62 nt upstream from the translational start codon. The *lef* gene has one apparent transcriptional start site at 29 nt upstream from the translational start codon. Regions with similarity to canonical sequences of *Bacillus subtilis* promoters are not apparent in the promoter regions of either gene (DAI et al. 1995).

Transcription of the *pagA* gene is more complex. *pagA* is the first gene of an autogenously controlled bicistronic operon (HOFFMASTER and KOEHLER 1999). The downstream gene, *pagR*, negatively controls expression of the *pag* operon. Cells producing PA have two mRNA transcripts corresponding to *pagA*: a short 2.7-kb transcript and a longer 4.2-kb transcript representing a bicistronic message derived from *pagA* and *pagR*. The 3′ end of the short transcript maps adjacent to an inverted repeat sequence between the two genes. Attenuation of termination at this site results in transcription of *pagR*. Steady-state levels of *pagA* mRNA are increased 2.5- to 7-fold in a *pagR* mutant. The mechanism for control of the operon by *pagR* is not known. No DNA-binding activity of the PagR protein has been reported. However, the predicted amino acid sequence of the putative PagR protein is similar to certain other regulatory proteins that contain helix-turn-helix motifs and are predicted to be DNA-binding proteins. The relatively weak activity of *pagR* may not be physiologically significant for *B. anthracis* virulence. In a mouse model for anthrax, the LD_{50} of a *pagR* mutant did not differ from that of the parent strain (HOFFMASTER and KOEHLER 1999).

Unlike the *cya* and *lef* transcripts, the 5′ ends of mRNAs corresponding to the *pag* operon map to two different sites, termed P1 and P2 (KOEHLER et al. 1994). The P1 site is located 58 nt upstream from the translational start codon and is not adjacent to consensus sequences associated with *Bacillus subtilis* promoters. P2 is located 26 nt upstream of the translational start codon and is adjacent to appropriately spaced consensus sequences corresponding to σ^A-dependent promoters of *B. subtilis*. In *B. subtilis*, σ^A RNA polymerase is required for transcription of housekeeping genes. Nevertheless, the steady-state level of transcripts beginning at P2 is relatively low in all growth conditions tested. In conditions favoring toxin synthesis, the majority of *pag* transcripts have 5′ ends mapping to the P1 site. Transcription from P1 is induced by the CO_2/bicarbonate signal and requires the presence of a *trans*-acting gene, *atxA*, as described below.

The *capB*, *capC*, *capA*, and *dep* genes appear to be arranged in an operon. However, data indicating a single transcript have not been reported. The four ORFs lie adjacent to one another on a 4.7-kb region of pXO2 (Uchida et al. 1993b; Makino et al. 1989). Sequence analysis of the intergenic regions, which range from 12 to 183 bp, does not indicate the presence of transcription terminators. mRNAs with 5′ ends mapping to two sites, P1 and P2, have been mapped to positions 731 bp and 625 bp, respectively, upstream of the translation initiation codon of *capB* (Uchida et al. 1997). Sequences upstream of the P1 site match poorly to the consensus sequence of *B. subtilis* σ^A-dependent promoters, and no appropriately spaced promoter consensus sequences are located upstream of P2. Data from quantitative analysis of primer extension products indicate that the steady-state level of transcripts mapping to P2 is approximately 40% of the level of P1 transcripts. Levels of both transcripts are regulated by *atxA* and *acpA* and are induced by CO_2/bicarbonate. It is not clear whether initiation of transcription begins at P2 or processing of P1 transcripts results in mRNAs with 5′ ends mapping to P2 (Uchida et al. 1997).

4 Plasmid-Encoded Virulence Gene Regulators

4.1 AtxA: A Unique Global Regulator

The pXO1-encoded gene *atxA* (anthrax toxin activator) is a global regulator of virulence gene expression in *B. anthracis*. *atxA*-deleted strains produce no detectable EF, LF, or PA and exhibit reduced capsule synthesis (Dai et al. 1995; Uchida et al. 1997; Guignot et al. 1997). The *atxA* gene was discovered by two groups independently. Uchida et al. (Uchida et al. 1993a) cloned *atxA* as a gene that stimulated expression of a *pag-lacZ* transcriptional fusion in a *B. subtilis* background. Koehler et al. (Koehler et al. 1994) identified *atxA* using transposon-mediated insertional mutagenesis. *Tn917-LTV3* insertion libraries of a $pXO1^+$ $pXO2^-$ strain were screened in an immunoassay for mutants that exhibited decreased PA synthesis. PA-deficient isolates contained transposon insertions that either disrupted the *pagA* gene or the *atxA* locus. Further investigations revealed that the 1.4-kb *atxA* gene is required for transcription of *cya*, *lef*, and the major (P1-initiated) *pagA* transcript (DAI et al. 1995). Although *atxA* is not required for transcription of the *cap* genes, *atxA* can increase levels of the P1 and P2 transcripts initiated upstream of *capB* (UCHIDA et al. 1997).

The mechanism by which *atxA* controls gene expression is not known. *atxA* encodes a basic soluble 56-kDa protein with no apparent structural motifs. Although *atxA* regulates CO_2/bicarbonate-induced genes, steady-state levels of *atxA* mRNA and protein are unaffected by CO_2/bicarbonate (DAI and KOEHLER 1997). The *atxA* gene appears to be expressed constitutively as a monocistronic transcript throughout growth in batch culture (T. Koehler, unpublished results). One apparent transcription initiation site has been reported for *atxA*, 99 bp upstream from the translational start site of the gene (DAI et al. 1995). Sequences indicating recognition sites for σ^A RNA polymerase are located upstream of this site. However, measurements of mRNA and protein indicate relatively low expression of the *atxA* gene in batch culture (DAI and KOEHLER 1997). Despite the apparent weak expression of *atxA*, AtxA levels do not appear to be limiting for toxin gene expression. Strains carrying multiple copies of the *pagA* promoter synthesize normal levels of PA (SIRARD et al. 1995). Moreover, a tenfold increase in *atxA* expression by a strain harboring *atxA* on a multicopy plasmid results in a slight decrease in PA levels (DAI and KOEHLER 1997).

atxA mutants are avirulent in a mouse model for anthrax, and *atxA*-null infected animals show a significantly decreased antibody response to all three toxin proteins (DAI et al. 1995). Therefore, *atxA* appears to regulate toxin gene expression during infection.

4.2
AcpA: A Capsule Gene-Specific Regulator

A second, more specific *trans*-acting regulator is located on pXO2. The *acpA* (anthrax capsule activator) gene encodes a *trans*-acting regulator that appears to be specific for expression of the capsule biosynthetic genes. *acpA* was discovered by Vietri et al. (VIETRI et al. 1995) after transposon mutagenesis of a $pXO1^-$ $pXO2^+$ *B. anthracis* strain. A Tn*917*-insertion mutant that produced rough colonies when grown in conditions appropriate for capsule synthesis harbored an 8.2-kb deletion outside of the *cap* gene region on pXO2. The *acpA* gene, located over 11 kb from the *cap* genes, complemented the capsule-deficient phenotype of the mutant when the gene was introduced *in trans* on a multicopy plasmid. Results of transcriptional analyses indicate that *acpA* is required for transcription of *capB*, the first gene of the apparent *cap* gene operon, in $pXO1^-$ $pXO2^+$ strains (Vietri et al. 1995). As is true for *atxA*, the mechanism by which *acpA* controls *cap* expression is not known.

4.3 Functional Similarities of *atxA* and *acpA*

The *atxA* and *acpA* genes were discovered and initially characterized in strains carrying single virulence plasmids: *atxA* as a regulator of the toxin structural genes (Uchida et al. 1993a; Koehler et al. 1994) and *acpA* as a regulator of the capsule biosynthetic genes (Vietri et al. 1995). Subsequent work revealed structural and functional similarities between the two regulators. The *atxA* and *acpA* genes encode proteins of comparable size (56 and 55 kDa, respectively), and the predicted amino acid sequences are 28% identical and 51% similar throughout. Sequence comparisons of AtxA and AcpA with other proteins in databases do not reveal potential homologues. It is notable, however, that the *B. anthracis* regulators are 47%–52% similar to a regulatory protein of *Streptococcus pyogenes*, Mga (for multigene activator). The Mga protein, which contains a helix-turn-helix motif, has been demonstrated to specifically bind target DNA sequences of certain virulence genes in *S. pyogenes* (McIver et al. 1995). However, the predicted amino acid sequences of AtxA and AcpA do not suggest DNA-binding ability, and sequence-specific interactions between the regulators and the promoter regions of target genes have not been demonstrated.

Considering that both regulators positively control expression of CO_2/bicarbonate-induced virulence genes, Uchida et al. (Uchida et al. 1997) tested *atxA* and *acpA* for functional homology. These investigators demonstrated that the *atxA* gene cloned on a multicopy plasmid in a $pXO1^-$ $pXO2^+$ strain activates expression of *capB* in the presence or absence of *acpA*. Yet *acpA* cloned on a multi-copy plasmid in a $pXO1^+$ $pXO2^-$ strain does not activate toxin gene expression. Thus there is unidirectional cross-talk between pXO1 and pXO2. The pXO1-encoded regulator *atxA* controls virulence genes on both plasmids, whereas the pXO2-encoded regulator *acpA* is specific for the capsule genes.

Further investigations are required to determine the relative contributions of *atxA* and *acpA* to capsule gene expression. Strains harboring pXO1 and pXO2 produce more capsule than strains carrying only pXO2 (GREEN et al. 1985), and the enhanced capsule synthesis by strains harboring both plasmids has been attributed to *atxA* (GUIGNOT et al. 1997). In a pXO1$^-$ pXO2$^+$ strain *acpA* mRNA levels are increased during growth in elevated CO_2/bicarbonate relative to growth in air (VIETRI et al. 1995), suggesting that AcpA levels are limiting for *cap* expression. In contrast, *atxA* mRNA and protein levels in pXO1$^+$ pXO2$^-$ cells are not affected by the CO_2/bicarbonate signal (DAI and KOEHLER 1997).

5
Growth Phase-Dependent Toxin Expression

When *B. anthracis* is grown in batch culture under optimal conditions for toxin synthesis the steady-state levels of toxin gene transcripts and toxin proteins are highest during the transition from exponential phase to stationary phase (KOEHLER et al. 1994; LEPPLA 1988, 1991; SIRARD et al. 1994). For an increasing number of bacteria, production of toxins and other virulence factors at the end of exponential growth when cells are at a high density has been attributed to quorum sensing. The individual cells of a bacterial population produce a diffusible signal molecule that, after crossing a concentration threshold, interacts with a histidine kinase sensor and a transcriptional activator to induce gene expression (DUNNY and WINANS 1999). To date, there are no reports of *B. anthracis* virulence gene control by quorum sensing. In all growth conditions tested in our laboratory, addition of cell-free, spent media to *B. anthracis* cultures did not affect toxin gene expression or expression of *atxA* (T. Koehler, unpublished data).

Growth phase-dependent toxin gene expression in *B. anthracis* is associated with *abrB*, an ortholog of a well-studied *B. subtilis* gene (SAILE and KOEHLER 2002). In *B. subtilis*, *abrB* has been termed a "transition state regulator" because it activates and represses numerous genes during transitions in growth phase, from lag to exponential and from exponential to stationary phase (STRAUCH 1993). The first evidence for *abrB*-controlled anthrax toxin gene expression was obtained by BAILLE et al. (BAILLIE et al. 1998), who demonstrated that a *B. subtilis abrB* mutant harboring *pagA* on a multicopy plasmid exhibited an eightfold increase in PA synthesis compared with the parent strain harboring the same plasmid construct.

Using the incomplete *B. anthracis* chromosome sequence database of The Institute for Genomic Research and the *B. anthracis* plasmid sequence databases, SAILE and KOEHLER (SAILE and KOEHLER 2002) identified two orthologs of the *B. subtilis abrB* gene in *B. anthracis*: one on the chromosome and one on pXO1. Deletion of the pXO1 *abrB* ortholog does not affect toxin gene expression. However, the *abrB* ortholog on the *B. anthracis* chromosome regulates expression of the three anthrax toxin genes.

The *B. anthracis* chromosome-encoded *abrB* represses the toxin genes and affects the timing of toxin gene expression in batch culture (SAILE and KOEHLER 2002). In *B. anthracis* strains harboring toxin gene promoter-*lacZ* fusions at the normal genetic loci, β-galactosidase activity increases gradually throughout exponential phase, reaching maximum activity in late exponential phase. In contrast, the enzyme activity of reporter strains deleted for *abrB* increases sharply in early exponential phase, reaching maximum activity in mid-exponential phase. Of the three toxin genes, *pagA* is the most strongly affected by *abrB*. Expression of a transcriptional *pagA-lacZ* fusion in the chromosomal *abrB* mutant is increased up to 20-fold during early exponential growth compared with the parent strain. *lef-lacZ* and *cya-lacZ* expression during early log phase growth increases only two- to threefold in the *abrB*-null mutant. Results of Western hybridization analysis indicate increased PA, LF, and EF synthesis in the absence of a functional *abrB* gene.

The chromosomal *abrB* gene of *B. anthracis* is predicted to encode a 94-amino acid protein that is 85% identical to *B. subtilis* AbrB (SAILE and KOEHLER 2002). The mechanism for AbrB-controlled toxin expression in *B. anthracis* is not yet known. In *B. subtilis*, AbrB has been shown to be a DNA-binding protein that controls over 40 different genes (STRAUCH 1993). A 16-bp AT-rich consensus sequence for AbrB binding has been proposed (STRAUCH 1995), and some potential binding sites can be found in the anthrax toxin gene promoter regions (BAILLIE et al. 1998). However, numerous sites can be found throughout the 67% AT *B. anthracis* genome, making predictions of specific DNA-binding sites somewhat unconvincing (SAILE and KOEHLER 2002).

The involvement of an *abrB* ortholog in the regulation of toxin synthesis in *Bacillus anthracis* ties anthrax toxin gene expression to the complex network of postexponential phase adaptive responses that have been well studied in *B. subtilis*. In *B. subtilis*, expression of the *abrB* gene is transient and highly growth phase dependent. Highest levels of *abrB* transcript and protein are found during the transition from lag phase into exponential growth (O'Reilly and Devine 1997). After this early peak, levels drop sharply because of negative regulation by the phosphorylated form of response regulator Spo0A (O'Reilly and Devine 1997; Strauch 1993). Although little is known regarding expression of *abrB* in *B. anthracis*, negative regulation by the *B. anthracis spo0A* gene has been reported (Saile and Koehler 2002).

6 Model for Virulence Gene Regulation

Data from genetic experiments employing strains with null-mutations in regulatory genes suggest a model for virulence gene control in which *atxA* is the central player, as shown in Fig. 1. Virulence gene expression has been compared in parent and mutant strains by measuring relative levels of *pagA*, *lef*, *cya*, and *capB* mRNAs; toxin proteins; and capsule material. Transcription of the toxin genes absolutely requires *atxA* (Dai et al. 1995), whereas *capB* transcription requires the presence of either *atxA* or *acpA*

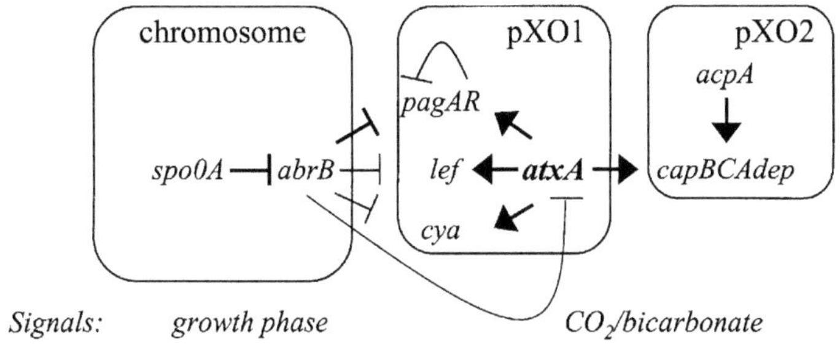

Fig. 1. Model for virulence gene regulation. Regulatory genes on the *B. anthracis* chromosome and the two virulence plasmids are shown. The pXO1 gene *atxA* positively regulates expression of the three anthrax toxin genes, *pagA*, *lef*, and *cya*, and *capB*, the first gene in an apparent operon that is required for capsule biosynthesis. The *lef* and *cya* genes are expressed as monocistronic transcripts, whereas the *pagA* gene is cotranscribed with *pagR*, a weak repressor of the *pag* operon. In addition to control by *atxA*, *cap* expression is positively regulated by the pXO2 gene *acpA*. Expression of *atxA*- and *acpA*-regulated genes is enhanced when cells are grown in certain media in the presence of elevated CO_2/bicarbonate. Growth phase-specific expression of the toxin genes is controlled by the chromosomal gene *abrB*. *abrB* exerts a strong negative effect on *pagA* and smaller effects on the other toxin genes and *atxA*. The chromosomal gene *spo0A* controls *abrB* expression. Direct interactions between regulatory proteins and DNA have not been demonstrated for any of the relationships indicated

(UCHIDA et al. 1997). The *pagA* gene is cotranscribed with *pagR*, a weak repressor that autogenously controls the *pag* operon (HOFFMASTER and KOEHLER 1999). Toxin and capsule gene transcription is greatest when cells are grown in defined media in elevated CO_2/bicarbonate (BARTKUS and LEPPLA 1989; CATALDI et al. 1992; KOEHLER et al. 1994; SIRARD et al. 1994; VIETRI et al. 1995). Interestingly, CO_2/bicarbonate increases expression of *acpA* (VIETRI et al. 1995), whereas *atxA* expression is unaffected (DAI and KOEHLER 1997). Growth phase-dependent toxin synthesis is associated with the chromosomal gene *abrB*. *abrB* represses expression of all three toxin genes, exerting its greatest effect during exponential growth. The *pag* operon is more strongly repressed by *abrB* than the *lef* or *cya* genes (SAILE and KOEHLER 2002).

Specific DNA-binding activity has not been demonstrated for any of the regulatory proteins. Genes that are coordinately expressed in response to the same signals or regulators often have sequence similarities in the promoter regions. The minimal upstream sequences required for activation of *pag* and *capB* have been determined (DAI et al. 1995; UCHIDA et al. 1997). Although direct sequence comparisons are difficult in *B. anthracis* because of the AT-rich nature of the genome, it is notable that examination of the promoter regions of *pag*, *capB*, and the other *atxA*-activated genes does not reveal obvious similarities in sequences or predicted secondary structures.

At present there are no candidates for *atxA*-regulated genes that act downstream of the global regulator to activate virulence gene expression. Hoffmaster and Koehler (HOFFMASTER and KOEHLER 1997) reported evidence of additional *atxA*-activated genes in a $pXO1^+$ $pXO2^-$ *B. anthracis* strain. However, none of these has been found to be involved in toxin gene expression. It has been proposed that AtxA interacts with another protein to mediate virulence gene activation (HOFFMASTER and KOEHLER 1997).

The relatively new discovery of *abrB*-controlled toxin gene expression implicates an additional level of control that may not be directly tied to *atxA*. A clear epistatic relationship between *abrB* and *atxA* has not been established. Although *abrB* has a small, approximately fourfold, negative effect on *atxA* expression (SAILE and KOEHLER 2002), steady-state levels of AtxA are not limiting for toxin gene expression (DAI and KOEHLER 1997). Thus the small effect of *abrB* on *atxA* expression cannot explain the differences in toxin gene expression observed in an *abrB* mutant. It is conceivable that in *B. anthracis*, *abrB* controls toxin gene expression directly or controls another unidentified regulator important for expression of one or more of the toxin genes. In *B. subtilis*, some of the effects of AbrB on gene expression are indirect, resulting from repression of additional regulatory genes by AbrB (STRAUCH 1993). Finally, the emergence of the *abrB* pathway reveals for the first time a differential effect of a regulator on the three toxin genes. The differences may be due to differing binding affinities of AbrB for the toxin gene promoters or may indicate divergent mechanisms for control of these genes.

7 Other Virulence Factors

Although the anthrax toxin proteins and capsule are considered to be the major virulence factors of the bacterium, other genes affect *B. anthracis* virulence. A germination operon located within the pXO1 pathogenicity island appears to play a role in germination of *B. anthracis* spores during infection (GUIDI-RONTANI et al. 1999a). The *gerX* operon (for germination pXO1-related) is comprised of *gerXB*, *gerXA*, and *gerXC*. The predicted products of the three genes are similar to proteins encoded by *ger* operons of *B. subtilis*, *cereus*, and *megaterium*. As is true for other germination operons, *gerX* transcription occurs during sporulation. Expression of *gerX* is associated with the forespore compartment after septation. This expression pattern is consistent with the presence of a consensus sequence for the forespore-specific RNA polymerase sigma factor σ^G upstream of the transcriptional start site for the operon.

A *gerX*-null mutant is less virulent than the parent strain in a mouse model (GUIDI-RONTANI et al. 1999a). Although the mechanism for attenuation of virulence is not clear, data indicate that the mutant strain germinates less efficiently in vivo and in vitro within macrophages. The rate of germination may have a strong effect on the fate of the infected host. It has been postulated that the *gerX*-encoded proteins are part of a unique system for detection of specific signals in the host environment and transduction of the signals into the *B. anthracis* spore.

Another gene that most likely has a role in adaptation of *B. anthracis* to the host environment is *sigB*. The *sigB* gene, well-characterized in *B. subtilis*, encodes the general stress transcription factor σ^B (HELMAN and MORAN 2002). In *B. subtilis*, σ^B RNA polymerase initiates transcription of over 100 genes that together comprise the σ^B regulon. Two orthologs of genes that are *sigB*-regulated in *B. subtilis* were identified in *B. anthracis*

(FOUET et al. 2000). The *B. anthracis* genes are induced during stationary phase and by heat shock. Specific functions of *sigB*-regulated genes in *B. anthracis* have not been examined. However, a *sigB* mutant is less virulent than the parental strain in a mouse model, indicating that the *B. anthracis* *sigB* gene may be a minor virulence factor.

8 Genetic Manipulation of *B. anthracis*

8.1 Strains Used in Genetic Studies

Attenuated *B. anthracis* strains designated Sterne and Pasteur have been used in most studies of virulence gene expression. The Sterne strain is a $pXO1^+$ $pXO2^-$ strain that currently serves as the live vaccine for use in animals. Strains 7702, Weybridge, and a colony variant of Weybridge, termed "Weybridge A" are all considered Sterne strains. The Pasteur strain is $pXO1^-$ $pXO2^+$. Two different strains, 4229 and 6602, have been called Pasteur. Despite the apparent lack of genetic variation in *B. anthracis* (see chapter 2 of this volume), these strains exhibit slight differences in growth rate, sporulation efficiency, colony morphology, and phage sensitivity.

8.2 DNA Exchange in *Bacillus* Species

Early studies of pXO1 and pXO2 were facilitated by the development of methods for genetic exchange between *Bacillus cereus* group species. The *B. anthracis* virulence plasmids are not self-transmissible, but they can be mobilized by certain conjugative plasmids originally found in *B. thuringiensis* subspecies *thuringiensis*. The most thoroughly studied of these is pXO12, a self-transmissible plasmid that can transfer pXO1, pXO2, and a small tetracycline resistance plasmid pBC16, in intra- and interspecies matings (BATTISTI et al. 1985; GREEN et al. 1989). *B. cereus* group species carrying pXO12 have been shown to transfer pBC16 at frequencies from 2×10^{-4} to 7×10^{-2} Tc^r transconjugants per donor. pXO12 carries no readily selectable markers but is associated with the ability of cells to synthesize parasporal crystals. In matings employing $pXO12^+$ $pBC16^+$ donors, Tc^r ($pBC16^+$) transconjugants can be screened for the presence of pXO12 by screening for donor ability or by examining cells microscopically for the presence of parasporal crystals. Frequencies of cotransfer of pXO12 with pBC16 vary depending on the donor-recipient pair, but in some experiments approach 80%.

Transfer of the virulence plasmids pXO1 and pXO2 by pXO12$^+$ *B. anthracis* strains occurs at low frequencies. When a pXO1$^+$ pXO12$^+$ pBC16$^+$ *B. anthracis* donor is mated with cured *B. anthracis* recipients, 0.3% of the Tc^r transconjugants also carry pXO1. A pXO2$^+$ pXO12$^+$ pBC16$^+$ *B. anthracis* donor transfers pXO2 to *B. cereus* at a similar frequency. Transfer of the virulence plasmids is thought to occur by conduction. Cointegrates of pXO12 and pXO1 involving the insertion element IS*4430* form in the donor strain and are resolved, sometimes improperly, in transconjugants (Green et al. 1989).

A conjugative system for transfer of plasmids from *B. subtilis* into *B. anthracis* has also been described but is less well-characterized than pXO12-mediated conjugation. Plasmid pLS20, originally found in *B. subtilis* (*natto*) is self-transmissible and can mobilize pBC16 and certain other small plasmids (Koehler and Thorne 1987) into a diverse group of *Bacillus* species. Transfer of pXO1 and pXO2 by pLS20 has not been reported.

Conjugative transfer of DNA into and out of *B. anthracis* is limited to plasmid DNA. However, transducing phage can transfer plasmids between *B. cereus* group species and chromosomal DNA between strains of the same species. Although a number of phages have been described, bacteriophage CP-51 is the most useful because it can package large amounts of DNA (Thorne 1993). CP-51-mediated transduction of pXO2 from *B. anthracis* to *B. cereus* was instrumental in demonstrating that the plasmid was associated with capsule synthesis (Green et al. 1985).

8.3 Construction of Recombinant Strains

More recently, advancement of methods to introduce foreign and recombinant DNA into *B. anthracis* has allowed further manipulation of the genome. Although *B. anthracis* is not transformable by methods commonly used for other Gram-positive organisms, certain plasmids can be electroporated into *B. anthracis* at frequencies up to 10^4 transformants per microgram of DNA (Koehler 2000). Vectors derived from a number of naturally occurring plasmids of other Gram-positive species, including pBC16, pE194, pC194, and pUB110, have been introduced into *B. anthracis* using electroporation. Electroporation frequencies are highest when plasmids are isolated from DNA methyltransferase-deficient (*dam*) *E. coli* strains or from *B. subtilis* 168, a strain that is not known to possess adenine methylating activities. These observations suggest that *B. anthracis* has a restriction system dependent on a specific pattern of adenine methylation for the recognition of foreign DNA (MARRERO and WELKOS 1995). There are no reports of electroporation of pXO1, pXO2, or linear DNA fragments into *B. anthracis*.

A recombinant conjugal system can also be used to transfer plasmids directly from *E. coli* to *B. anthracis*. Shuttle vectors containing replication origins and selectable markers functional in both species and the transfer origin of the IncP plasmid RK2 can be mobilized by self-transmissible IncP plasmids coresident in *E. coli* donors (TRIEU-CUOT et al. 1991).

Introduction of specific delivery vectors into *B. anthracis* with electroporation or conjugal transfer has facilitated construction of *B. anthracis* mutants harboring specific insertions and gene replacements. A delivery vector harboring a selectable marker flanked by *B. anthracis* DNA homologous to the target locus can be constructed in *E. coli*. On introduction of the construct into *B. anthracis*, homologous recombination between the vector-borne DNA and the *B. anthracis* genome results in creation of a mutant strain.

Three types of delivery vectors have been used to create mutants. The naturally occurring *B. subtilis* plasmid pE194 is temperature-sensitive for replication. pE194-derived constructs carrying *B. anthracis* DNA sequences can be electroporated into *B. anthracis* with initial selection at 32 °C, the permissive temperature. Mutants carrying the plasmid inserted into the *B. anthracis* genome can be isolated after growth at 43 °C with selection for the plasmid-encoded *erm* gene (BROWN et al. 1994). Unfortunately, use of this vector is not very efficient because *B. anthracis* will not grow at temperatures exceeding 43 °C, and incomplete curing of pE194-derived vectors is observed at this temperature.

A second delivery vector is the *E. coli-B. anthracis* shuttle plasmid pUTE29. Derivatives of pUTE29 can be electroporated into *B. anthracis* with selection for the plasmid-encoded tetracycline-resistance marker. However, the plasmid is readily lost from *B. anthracis* in the absence of selection. When DNA sequences flanking a *B. anthracis* gene are cloned flanking a second selectable marker in pUTE29, the marker can be introduced into the *B. anthracis* genome by a double-crossover recombination event. This method has been particularly useful for construction of strains deleted for specific genes (DAI et al. 1995).

Finally, integrative vectors, carrying *B. anthracis* DNA sequences and lacking a replication origin functional in *B. anthracis*, can be transferred from *E. coli* to *B. anthracis* with selection for plasmid-encoded markers with the RK2 mating system. This strategy was used to disrupt each of the anthrax toxin genes on pXO1 and to create transcriptional fusions of toxin and capsule gene promoters to the β-galactosidase gene *lacZ*, creating important strains for studies of toxin gene expression and function (PEZARD et al. 1991; SIRARD et al. 1994).

8.4
Random Mutagenesis

Transposons Tn*916* and Tn*917*, from *Enterococcus faecalis*, have been employed for insertional mutagenesis in *B. anthracis*. Although transposon mutagenesis has resulted in the discovery of important genes, including the virulence gene regulators *atxA* and *acpA* (UCHIDA et al. 1993a; KOEHLER et al. 1994; VIETRI et al. 1995), neither transposon is ideal. Tn*916* insertion mutants are unstable in the absence of selection for the tetracycline-resistance gene encoded by the transposon (IVINS et al. 1990). Tn*917*-insertion mutants appear to be stable, yet insertion of this transposon is often accompanied by local deletions and rearrangements of *B. anthracis* DNA (KOEHLER et al. 1994). Moreover, in *B. anthracis* strains harboring either pXO1 or pXO2, Tn*917* appears to transpose preferentially to the virulence plasmids relative to the chromosome (HOFFMASTER and KOEHLER 1997). The apparent high frequency of transposon insertions on the plasmids may actually be the result of homologous recombination between transposon sequences and numerous insertion sequence-like elements on the plasmids.

Point mutants of *B. anthracis* can be isolated after UV mutagenesis of spores. Rifampicin- and streptomycin-resistant mutants and numerous amino acid, purine, and pyrimidine auxotrophs have been obtained by this method (BATTISTI et al. 1985). Unfortunately, low electroporation and *E. coli-B. anthracis* mating frequencies make it difficult to screen genomic libraries for clones that complement point mutants, making mapping of point mutations difficult.

9
Future Directions

Although knowledge of toxin and capsule gene expression by *B. anthracis* growing in batch culture is steadily increasing, studies of virulence gene expression by *B. anthracis* growing in the host have been limited. Anthrax infections generally begin with entry of *B. anthracis* spores into the gastrointestinal tract, the lungs, or the skin. Vegetative bacilli proliferate, spread systemically, and produce the capsule and secrete the anthrax toxin proteins. The timing and location of toxin and capsule synthesis by *B. anthracis* during infection are not clear. Germination of *B. anthracis* spores in alveolar murine macrophages after infection by the respiratory route has been reported (GUIDI-RONTANI et al. 1999b) (see chapter 6 of this volume). Newly germinated vegetative cells appear to express the toxin genes and *atxA* within the macrophage. However, it is not known whether expression of these genes before extracellular proliferation of the bacterium is significant for anthrax disease. Comparison of the LD_{50} values for various mutants in animal models provides important but limited information. Future investigations should address control of virulence gene expression in the changing environment of the host.

Genetic approaches have revealed key regulatory genes for toxin and capsule synthesis, yet the mechanisms by which the regulatory proteins control target genes are not known. To date, no protein-nucleic acid or protein-protein interactions have been reported. Moreover, the molecular bases for the effects of elevated CO_2/bicarbonate and temperature on virulence gene expression have not been determined. One of the most intriguing questions concerns the apparent redundancy in *atxA* and *acpA* function with regard to capsule synthesis. The relative contributions of *atxA* and *acpA* to capsule gene expression is not clear for *B. anthracis* growing in or out of the host. The discovery of *abrB*-controlled toxin synthesis links virulence gene expression to the multicomponent phosphorelay signaling system, well studied in *B. subtilis*. Yet it is not known whether this signaling system plays a role in environmental sensing by *B. anthracis* during infection.

Certainly there are important players in *B. anthracis* virulence regulation that are yet to be discovered. Further advances in genetic approaches for investigations of gene expression in this organism will facilitate identification and characterization of these factors. Improved transposon mutagenesis, a tightly controlled inducible promoter system, and a method for counterselection of genes would all be welcome additions to the current repertoire of genetic tools for *B. anthracis*. The availability of the incomplete genome sequence has already facilitated construction of specific mutants. Soon, DNA microarray analyses will allow screens for additional targets of transcriptional regulators that may be important in anthrax disease. Annotation and comparative analysis of the genome sequence will lead to new hypotheses that can be tested with the growing *B. anthracis* genetic toolbox.

References

Baillie L, Moir A, Manchee R (1998) The expression of the protective antigen of *Bacillus anthracis* in *Bacillus subtilis*. J Appl Microbiol 84:741–746

Bartkus JM, Leppla SH (1989) Transcriptional regulation of the protective antigen gene of *Bacillus anthracis*. Infect Immun 57:2295–2300

Battisti L, Green BD, Thorne CB (1985) Mating system for transfer of plasmids among *Bacillus anthracis*, *Bacillus cereus*, and *Bacillus thuringiensis*. J Bacteriol 162: 543–550

Bragg TS, Robertson DL (1989) Nucleotide sequence and analysis of the lethal factor gene (*lef*) from *Bacillus anthracis*. Gene 81:45–54

Brown DP, Ganova-Raeva L, Green BD, Wilkinson SR, Young M, Youngman P (1994) Characterization of *spo0A* homologues in diverse *Bacillus* and *Clostridium* species identifies a probable DNA-binding domain. Mol Microbiol 14:411–426

Cataldi A, Fouet A, Mock M (1992) Regulation of *pag* gene expression in *Bacillus anthracis*: use of a *pag-lacZ* transcriptional fusion. FEMS Microbiol Lett 98: 89–94

Dai Z, Koehler TM. (1997) Regulation of anthrax toxin activator gene (*atxA*) expression in *Bacillus anthracis*: Temperature, not CO_2/bicarbonate, affects AtxA synthesis. Infect Immun 65:2576–2582

Dai Z, Sirard J-C, Mock M, Koehler TM (1995) The *atxA* gene product activates transcription of the anthrax toxin genes and is essential for virulence. Mol Microbiol 16:1171–1181

Dunny GM, Winans SC (1999) Cell-cell signaling in bacteria. Washington, DC: ASM Press

Fouet A, Namy O, Lambert G (2000) Characterization of the operon encoding the alternative sigma(B) factor from *Bacillus anthracis* and its role in virulence. J Bacteriol 182:5036–5045

Fouet A, Sirard JC, Mock M (1994) *Bacillus anthracis* pXO1 virulence plasmid encodes a type 1 DNA topoisomerase. Mol Microbiol 11:471–479

Green BD, Battisti L, Koehler TM, Thorne CB (1985) Demonstration of a capsule plasmid in *Bacillus anthracis*. Infect Immun 49:291–297

Green BD, Battisti L, Thorne CB (1989) Involvement of Tn4430 in transfer of *Bacillus anthracis* plasmids mediated by *Bacillus thuringiensis* plasmid pXO12. J Bacteriol 171:104–113

Guidi-Rontani C, Pereira Y, Ruffie S, Sirard JC, Weber-Levy M, Mock M (1999a) Identification and characterization of a germination operon on the virulence plasmid pXO1 of *Bacillus anthracis.* Mol Microbiol 33:407–414

Guidi-Rontani C, Weber-Levy M, Labruyere E, Mock M (1999b) Germination of *Bacillus anthracis* spores within alveolar macrophages. Mol Microbiol 31:9–17

Guignot J, Mock M, Fouet A (1997) AtxA activates the transcription of genes harbored by both *Bacillus anthracis* virulence plasmids. FEMS Microbiol Lett 147:203–207

Helman JD, Moran CP (2002) RNA polymerase and sigma factors. In: *Bacillus subtilis and its close relatives.* Sonenshein AL, Hoch JA and Losick R (eds) Washington, DC: ASM Press, pp. 289–312

Hoffmaster AR, Koehler TM (1997) The anthrax toxin activator gene *atxA* is associated with CO_2-enhanced non-toxin gene expression in *Bacillus anthracis.* Infect Immun 65:3091–3099

Hoffmaster AR, Koehler TM (1999) Autogenous regulation of the *Bacillus anthracis* pag operon. J Bacteriol 181:4485–4492

Ivins BE, Welkos SL, Knudson GB, Little SF (1990) Immunization against anthrax with aromatic compound-dependent (Aro^-) mutants of *Bacillus anthracis* and with recombinant strains of *Bacillus subtilis* that produce anthrax protective antigen. Infect Immun 58:303–308

Koehler TM (2000) *Bacillus anthracis.* In: Gram-positive pathogens. Fischetti VA, Novick RP, Ferretti JJ, Protnoy DA and Rood JI (eds) Washington, DC: ASM Press, pp 519–528

Koehler TM, Dai Z, Kaufman-Yarbray M (1994) Regulation of the *Bacillus anthracis* protective antigen gene: CO_2 and a *trans*-acting element activate transcription from one of two promoters. J Bacteriol 176:586–595

Koehler TM, Thorne CB (1987) *Bacillus subtilis* (*natto*) plasmid pLS20 mediates interspecies plasmid transfer. J Bacteriol 169:5271–5278

Leppla SH (1988) Production and purification of anthrax toxin. Methods Enzymol 165:103–116

Leppla SH (1991) Purification and characterization of adenylyl cyclase from *Bacillus anthracis.* Methods Enzymol 195:153–168

Makino S, Sasakawa C, Uchida I, Terakado N, Yoshikawa M (1988) Cloning and CO_2-dependent expression of the genetic region for encapsulation from *Bacillus anthracis.* Mol Microbiol 2:371–376

Makino S-I, Uchida I, Terakado N, Sasakawa C, Yoshikawa M (1989) Molecular characterization and protein analysis of the *cap* region, which is essential for encapsulation in *Bacillus anthracis.* J Bacteriol 171:722–730

Marrero R, Welkos SL (1995) The transformation frequency of plasmids into *Bacillus anthracis* is affected by adenine methylation. Gene 152:75–78

McIver KS, Heath AS, Green BD, Scott JR (1995) Specific binding of the activator Mga to promoter sequences of the *emm* and *scpA* genes in the group A streptococcus. J Bacteriol 177:6619–6624

Mikesell P, Ivins BE, Ristroph JD, Dreier TM (1983) Evidence for plasmid-mediated toxin production in *Bacillus anthracis.* Infect Immun 39:371–376

Mock M, Labruyere E, Glaser P, Danchin A, Ullmann A (1988) Cloning and expression of the calmodulin-sensitive *Bacillus anthracis* adenylate cyclase in *Escherichia coli.* Gene 64:277–284

OKINAKA RT, CLOUD K, HAMPTON O, HOFFMASTER A, HILL KK, KEIM P, KOEHLER TM, LAMKE G, KUMANO S, MAHILLON J, MANTER D, MARTINEZ Y, RICKE D, SVENSSON R, JACKSON PJ (1999) The sequence and organization of pXO1, the large *Bacillus anthracis* plasmid harboring the anthrax toxin genes. J Bacteriol 181:6509–6515

O'REILLY M, DEVINE KM (1997) Expression of AbrB, a transition state regulator from *Bacillus subtilis*, is growth phase dependent in a manner resembling that of Fis, the nucleoid binding protein from *Escherichia coli*. J Bacteriol 179:522–529

PEZARD C, BERCHE P, MOCK M (1991) Contribution of individual toxin components to virulence of *Bacillus anthracis*. Infect Immun 59:3472–3477

ROBERTSON DL, BRAGG TS, SIMPSON S, KASPAR R, XIE W, TIPPETTS MT (1990) Mapping and characterization of *Bacillus anthracis* plasmids pXO1 and pXO2. Salisbury Med Bull 68 (Spec Suppl): 55–58

ROBERTSON DL, TIPPETTS MT, LEPPLA SH (1988) Nucleotide sequence of the *Bacillus anthracis* edema factor gene (*cya*): a calmodulin-dependent adenylate cyclase. Gene 73:363–371

SAILE E, KOEHLER TM (2002) Control of anthrax toxin gene expression by the transition state regulator *abrB*. J Bacteriol 184:370–380

SIRARD J-C, MOCK M, FOUET A (1994) The three *Bacillus anthracis* toxin genes are coordinately regulated by bicarbonate and temperature. J Bacteriol 176:5188–5192

SIRARD J-C, MOCK M, FOUET A (1995) Molecular tools for the study of transcriptional regulation in *Bacillus anthracis*. Res Microbiol 146:729–737

STRAUCH MA (1993) Abr, a transition state regulator. In: *Bacillus subtilis* and other gram-positive bacteria. Sonenshein AL, Hoch JA and Losick R (eds) Washington, DC: ASM Press, pp 757–764

STRAUCH MA (1995) Delineation of AbrB-binding sites on the *Bacillus subtilis spo0H, kinB, ftsAZ*, and *pbpE* promoters and use of a derived homology to identify a previously unsuspected binding site in the *bsuB1* methylase promoter. J Bacteriol 177: 6999–7002

THORNE CB (1993) *Bacillus anthracis*. In: *Bacillus subtilis* and Other Gram-Positive Bacteria: Biochemistry, Physiology, and Molecular Genetics. Sonenshein AL, Hoch JA and Losick R (eds) Washington, DC: American Society for Microbiology, pp 113–124

TIPPETTS MT, ROBERTSON DL (1988) Molecular cloning and expression of the *Bacillus anthracis* edema factor toxin gene: a calmodulin-dependent adenylate cyclase. J Bacteriol 170:2263–2266

TRIEU-CUOT P, CARLIER C, POYART-SALMERON C, COURVALIN P (1991) Shuttle vectors containing a multiple cloning site and a *lacZ* alpha gene for conjugal transfer of DNA from *Escherichia coli* to gram-positive bacteria. *Gene* 102:99–104

UCHIDA I, HASHIMOTO K, MAKINO S, SASAKAWA C, YOSHIKAWA M, TERAKADO N (1987) Restriction map of a capsule plasmid of *Bacillus anthracis*. Plasmid 18:178–181

UCHIDA I, HORNUNG JM, THORNE CB, KLIMPEL KR, and LEPPLA SH (1993a) Cloning and characterization of a gene whose product is a *trans*-activator of anthracis toxin synthesis. J Bacteriol 175:5329–5338

UCHIDA I, MAKINO S, SASAKAWA C, YOSHIKAWA M, SUGIMOTO C, TERAKADO N (1993b) Identification of a novel gene, *dep*, associated with depolymerization of the capsular polymer in *Bacillus anthracis*. Mol Microbiol 9:487–496

Uchida I, Makino S, Sekizaki T, Terakado N (1997) Cross-talk to the genes for *Bacillus anthracis* capsule synthesis by *atxA*, the gene encoding the *trans*-activator of anthrax toxin synthesis. Mol Microbiol 23:1229–1240

Uchida I, Sekizaki T, Hashimoto K, Terakado N (1985) Association of encapsulation of *Bacillus anthracis* with a 60 megadalton plasmid. J Gen Microbiol 131: 363–367

Vietri NJ, Marrero R, Hoover TA, Welkos SL (1995) Identification and characterization of a *trans*-activator involved in the regulation of encapsulation by *Bacillus anthracis*. Gene 152:1–9

Vodkin MH, Leppla SH (1983) Cloning of the protective antigen gene of *Bacillus anthracis*. Cell 34:693–697

Welkos SL, Lowe JR, Eden-McCutchan F, Vodkin M, Leppla SH, Schmidt JJ (1988) Sequence and analysis of the DNA encoding protective antigen of *Bacillus anthracis*. Gene 69:287–300

Subject Index

Current Topics in Microbiology and Immunology

Volumes published since 1998 (and still available)

Vol. 228: **Pawson, Anthony I. (Ed.):** Protein Modules in Signal Transduction. 1998. 42 figs. IX, 368 pp. ISBN 3-540-63396-0

Vol. 229: **Kelsoe, Garnett; Flajnik, Martin (Eds.):** Somatic Diversification of Immune Responses. 1998. 38 figs. IX, 221 pp. ISBN 3-540-63608-0

Vol. 230: **Kärre, Klas; Colonna, Marco (Eds.):** Specificity, Function, and Development of NK Cells. 1998. 22 figs. IX, 248 pp. ISBN 3-540-63941-1

Vol. 231: **Holzmann, Bernhard; Wagner, Hermann (Eds.):** Leukocyte Integrins in the Immune System and Malignant Disease. 1998. 40 figs. XIII, 189 pp. ISBN 3-540-63609-9

Vol. 232: **Whitton, J. Lindsay (Ed.):** Antigen Presentation. 1998. 11 figs. IX, 244 pp. ISBN 3-540-63813-X

Vol. 233/I: **Tyler, Kenneth L.; Oldstone, Michael B. A. (Eds.):** Reoviruses I. 1998. 29 figs. XVIII, 223 pp. ISBN 3-540-63946-2

Vol. 233/II: **Tyler, Kenneth L.; Oldstone, Michael B. A. (Eds.):** Reoviruses II. 1998. 45 figs. XVI, 187 pp. ISBN 3-540-63947-0

Vol. 234: **Frankel, Arthur E. (Ed.):** Clinical Applications of Immunotoxins. 1999. 16 figs. IX, 122 pp. ISBN 3-540-64097-5

Vol. 235: **Klenk, Hans-Dieter (Ed.):** Marburg and Ebola Viruses. 1999. 34 figs. XI, 225 pp. ISBN 3-540-64729-5

Vol. 236: **Kraehenbuhl, Jean-Pierre; Neutra, Marian R. (Eds.):** Defense of Mucosal Surfaces: Pathogenesis, Immunity and Vaccines. 1999. 30 figs. IX, 296 pp. ISBN 3-540-64730-9

Vol. 237: **Claesson-Welsh, Lena (Ed.):** Vascular Growth Factors and Angiogenesis. 1999. 36 figs. X, 189 pp. ISBN 3-540-64731-7

Vol. 238: **Coffman, Robert L.; Romagnani, Sergio (Eds.):** Redirection of Th1 and Th2 Responses. 1999. 6 figs. IX, 148 pp. ISBN 3-540-65048-2

Vol. 239: **Vogt, Peter K.; Jackson, Andrew O. (Eds.):** Satellites and Defective Viral RNAs. 1999. 39 figs. XVI, 179 pp. ISBN 3-540-65049-0

Vol. 240: **Hammond, John; McGarvey, Peter; Yusibov, Vidadi (Eds.):** Plant Biotechnology. 1999. 12 figs. XII, 196 pp. ISBN 3-540-65104-7

Vol. 241: **Westblom, Tore U.; Czinn, Steven J.; Nedrud, John G. (Eds.):** Gastroduodenal Disease and Helicobacter pylori. 1999. 35 figs. XI, 313 pp. ISBN 3-540-65084-9

Vol. 242: **Hagedorn, Curt H.; Rice, Charles M. (Eds.):** The Hepatitis C Viruses. 2000. 47 figs. IX, 379 pp. ISBN 3-540-65358-9

Vol. 243: **Famulok, Michael; Winnacker, Ernst-L.; Wong, Chi-Huey (Eds.):** Combinatorial Chemistry in Biology. 1999. 48 figs. IX, 189 pp. ISBN 3-540-65704-5

Vol. 244: **Daëron, Marc; Vivier, Eric (Eds.):** Immunoreceptor Tyrosine-Based Inhibition Motifs. 1999. 20 figs. VIII, 179 pp. ISBN 3-540-65789-4

Vol. 245/I: **Justement, Louis B.; Siminovitch, Katherine A. (Eds.):** Signal Transduction and the Coordination of B Lymphocyte Development and Function I. 2000. 22 figs. XVI, 274 pp. ISBN 3-540-66002-X

Vol. 245/II: **Justement, Louis B.; Siminovitch, Katherine A. (Eds.):** Signal Transduction on the Coordination of B Lymphocyte Development and Function II. 2000. 13 figs. XV, 172 pp. ISBN 3-540-66003-8

Vol. 246: **Melchers, Fritz; Potter, Michael (Eds.):** Mechanisms of B Cell Neoplasia 1998. 1999. 111 figs. XXIX, 415 pp. ISBN 3-540-65759-2

Vol. 247: **Wagner, Hermann (Ed.):** Immunobiology of Bacterial CpG-DNA. 2000. 34 figs. IX, 246 pp. ISBN 3-540-66400-9

Vol. 248: **du Pasquier, Louis; Litman, Gary W. (Eds.):** Origin and Evolution of the Vertebrate Immune System. 2000. 81 figs. IX, 324 pp. ISBN 3-540-66414-9

Vol. 249: **Jones, Peter A.; Vogt, Peter K. (Eds.):** DNA Methylation and Cancer. 2000. 16 figs. IX, 169 pp. ISBN 3-540-66608-7

Vol. 250: **Aktories, Klaus; Wilkins, Tracy, D. (Eds.):** Clostridium difficile. 2000. 20 figs. IX, 143 pp. ISBN 3-540-67291-5

Vol. 251: **Melchers, Fritz (Ed.):** Lymphoid Organogenesis. 2000. 62 figs. XII, 215 pp. ISBN 3-540-67569-8

Vol. 252: **Potter, Michael; Melchers, Fritz (Eds.):** B1 Lymphocytes in B Cell Neoplasia. 2000. XIII, 326 pp. ISBN 3-540-67567-1

Vol. 253: **Gosztonyi, Georg (Ed.):** The Mechanisms of Neuronal Damage in Virus Infections of the Nervous System. 2001. approx. XVI, 270 pp. ISBN 3-540-67617-1

Vol. 254: **Privalsky, Martin L. (Ed.):** Transcriptional Corepressors. 2001. 25 figs. XIV, 190 pp. ISBN 3-540-67569-8

Vol. 255: **Hirai, Kanji (Ed.):** Marek's Disease. 2001. 22 figs. XII, 294 pp. ISBN 3-540-67798-4

Vol. 256: **Schmaljohn, Connie S.; Nichol, Stuart T. (Eds.):** Hantaviruses. 2001, 24 figs. XI, 196 pp. ISBN 3-540-41045-7

Vol. 257: **van der Goot, Gisou (Ed.):** Pore-Forming Toxins, 2001. 19 figs. IX, 166 pp. ISBN 3-540-41386-3

Vol. 258: **Takada, Kenzo (Ed.):** Epstein-Barr Virus and Human Cancer. 2001. 38 figs. IX, 233 pp. ISBN 3-540-41506-8

Vol. 259: **Hauber, Joachim, Vogt, Peter K. (Eds.):** Nuclear Export of Viral RNAs. 2001. 19 figs. IX, 131 pp. ISBN 3-540-41278-6

Vol. 260: **Burton, Didier R. (Ed.):** Antibodies in Viral Infection. 2001. 51 figs. IX, 309 pp. ISBN 3-540-41611-0

Vol. 261: **Trono, Didier (Ed.):** Lentiviral Vectors. 2002. 32 figs. X, 258 pp. ISBN 3-540-42190-4

Vol. 262: **Oldstone, Michael B.A. (Ed.):** Arenaviruses I. 2002, 30 figs. XVIII, 197 pp. ISBN 3-540-42244-7

Vol. 263: **Oldstone, Michael B. A. (Ed.):** Arenaviruses II. 2002, 49 figs. XVIII, 268 pp. ISBN 3-540-42705-8

Vol. 264/I: **Hacker, Jörg; Kaper, James B. (Eds.):** Pathogenicity Islands and the Evolution of Microbes. 2002. 34 figs. XVIII, 232 pp. ISBN 3-540-42681-7

Vol. 264/II: **Hacker, Jörg; Kaper, James B. (Eds.):** Pathogenicity Islands and the Evolution of Microbes. 2002. 24 figs. XVIII, 228 pp. ISBN 3-540-42682-5

Vol. 265: **Dietzschold, Bernhard; Richt, Jürgen A. (Eds.):** Protective and Pathological Immune Responses in the CNS. 2002. 21 figs. X, 278 pp. ISBN 3-540-42668-X

Vol. 266: **Cooper, Koproski (Eds.):** The Interface Between Innate and Acquired Immunity, 2002, 15 figs. XIV, 116 pp. ISBN 3-540-42894-1

Vol. 267: **Mackenzie, John S.; Barrett, Alan D. T.; Deubel, Vincent (Eds.):** Japanese Encephalitis and West Nile Viruses. 2002. 66 figs. X, 418 pp. ISBN 3-540-42783-X

Vol. 268: **Zwickl, Peter; Baumeister, Wolfgang (Eds.):** The Proteasome-Ubiquitin Protein Degradation Pathway. 2002, 17 figs. X, 213 pp. ISBN 3-540-43096-2

Vol. 269: **Koszinowski, Ulrich H.; Hengel, Hartmut (Eds.):** Viral Proteins Counteracting Host Defenses. 2002, 47 figs. XII, 325 pp. ISBN 3-540-43261-2

Vol. 270: **Beutler, Bruce; Wagner, Herrmann (Eds.):** Toll-Like Receptor Family Members and Their Ligands. 2002, 31 figs. X, approx. 212 pp. ISBN 3-540-43560-3

GPSR Compliance

The European Union's (EU) General Product Safety Regulation (GPSR) is a set of rules that requires consumer products to be safe and our obligations to ensure this.

If you have any concerns about our products, you can contact us on ProductSafety@springernature.com

In case Publisher is established outside the EU, the EU authorized representative is:

Springer Nature Customer Service Center GmbH
Europaplatz 3
69115 Heidelberg, Germany

Batch number: 10755332

Printed by Printforce, the Netherlands